Endoscopy in Pediatric Inflammatory Bowel Disease

Luigi Dall'Oglio · Claudio Romano
Editors

Endoscopy in Pediatric Inflammatory Bowel Disease

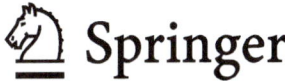

Springer

Editors
Luigi Dall'Oglio
Digestive Surgery and Endoscopic Unit
Bambino Gesù Children's Hospital
Rome, Italy

Claudio Romano
Gastroentology Unit, Pediatric Department
University of Messina
Messina, Italy

ISBN 978-3-030-09659-5   ISBN 978-3-319-61249-2   (eBook)
https://doi.org/10.1007/978-3-319-61249-2

Printed on acid-free paper

This Springer imprint is published by the registered company Springer International Publishing AG part of Springer Nature
The registered company address is: Gewerbestrasse 11, 6330 Cham, Switzerland

Foreword

Since its introduction in the late 1960s, the field of pediatric gastroenterology and endoscopy has developed rapidly. During the last 30 years, the number of pediatric gastroenterologists performing endoscopic procedures has progressively increased with pediatric endoscopy evolving from an infrequent procedure in the operating room to a routine outpatient procedure. The rapid growth and standardization of endoscopic procedures in children has been associated with an improvement of diagnosis and management of pediatric population with IBD. With approximately 25% of IBDs presenting before the patient is 20 years of age, pediatric endoscopy has become an integral part of a diagnostic process in a significant number of young IBD patients. Presentations in the pediatric population may differ from those typically seen in adults. Unique features in children may include growth failure and pubertal delay, which must be considered when planning treatment. Moreover, clear diagnosis of IBD and differentiation of CD from UC and/or IC are essential for pediatric patients in planning the optimal treatment strategy in a given patient. This is why endoscopy in this subset of population is very peculiar and requires dedicated skills and specific approaches which somehow may differ from those routinely used in adult IBD patients. Recommendations from the European and North American pediatric gastroenterology societies have helped to bring uniformity in the diagnostic work-up and the differentiation of IBD types. Nonetheless, a lot remains to be done to upgrade and standardize practice of pediatric endoscopy in the management of IBD populations. For the new generation of pediatric endoscopists, the challenge will be to properly use invasive endoscopic tests in association with noninvasive diagnostic tools like wireless capsule or fecal calprotectin. This makes imperative that gastroenterologists managing pediatric patients with IBD have a specific training path and develop extensive expertise for advanced diagnostic modalities including endoscopy of the small bowel such as enteroscopy. I am very pleased to introduce this very comprehensive and updated book dealing with the different topics of pediatric endoscopy in the field of IBD conditions. Every single chapter has been developed to provide the most extensive and practical guide to perform endoscopy according to the most recent guideline. All different aspects of IBD endoscopy are nicely discussed with a clinical approach where endoscopy is integrated as part of the instrumental and clinical framework required to provide early diagnosis and to guide therapy. The book reads really well and may represent a useful tool also for those pediatric gastroenterologists who are developing their training in endoscopy and have to quickly find the resources and the information to implement their endoscopic procedures in children with IBD. I do believe that the authors should be congratulated for this excellent piece of work, which will remain as one of the best available educational books for those who need an updated and extensive guide to support their practice in endoscopy for pediatric patients diagnosed with inflammatory conditions of the GI tract.

Milan, Italy   Alessandro Repici

Preface

Endoscopy can be considered an essential part of proper care in children with inflammatory bowel diseases (IBDs), including ulcerative colitis (UC) and Crohn's disease (CD). The role ranges widely from diagnosing the disease to assessing the extent of the disease and its activity. Major advances in recent years, with the emergence of new techniques such as wireless video capsule endoscopy (WCE), device-assisted enteroscopy (DAE), chromoendoscopy, and confocal endomicroscopy, have been achieved. In pediatric population, endoscopy has a major role in the differential diagnosis of the IBD, between CD and UC or indeterminate colitis. The techniques of sedation allow the execution of the exams with better safety. Endoscopic reassessment is considered in cases of frequent relapses, refractoriness, surgery, and in monitoring biological therapies response. The role of endoscopy in IBD is to assist in the diagnosis of IBD disease activity, in defines disease distribution/extent and assessment of treatment success (mucosal healing). Recently, new guidelines for endoscopy in IBD were published by the European Crohn's and Colitis Organization, but few details are available for pediatric specificity. In this book, we have summarized the main topics of endoscopy in pediatric inflammatory bowel disease as equipment in pediatric endoscopy, patient and parents preparation, sedation, endoscopic features in early onset IBD, esophagogastroduodenoscopy and ileocolonoscopy, application of the endoscopic scores, small bowel endoscopy, endoscopic intervention in IBD, and cancer and dysplasia surveillance. The selected authors have maximum competence in this field, and this book can be an important aid in clinical practice and in the management of children with IBD. We confirm that endoscopy is an important tool in the diagnosis and management of IBD, but the sensitivity and specificity are increased if this technique is used by expert hands and with proper interpretation of the results.

Messina, Italy   Claudio Romano

Contents

Equipment in Pediatric Endoscopy

1

Maria Teresa Illiceto, Gabriele Lisi, and Giuliano Lombardi

1.1 Introduction

The endoscopic techniques used in children are quite similar to those used in the adult. The anatomical differences, especially in children below 10–15 kg of body weight, condition the endoscopist while choosing the instrument:

- the newborn's esophagus measures 8–10 cm in length and approximately 5 mm in diameter, and the soft posterior wall of the trachea is easily compressed during upper endoscopy.
- in small children, the antrum is acutely angulated, requiring a greater degree of tip deflection to view the pylorus.
- in the same way, the proximal duodenum is angulated, obscuring views of the posteromedial wall [1].
- the diameter of the empty duodenum, jejunum, and ileum in newborns measure 10–15 mm.
- the neonatal colonic diameter is approximately 10 mm except for the cecum, that is approximately 17 mm.

An additional limitation to the choice of endoscopes diameter is the compression of the trachea with an endotracheal tube inside. Current technology permits safe visualization, tissue sampling, and therapeutic interventions of the upper and lower

M. T. Illiceto · G. Lombardi (✉)
Pediatric Digestive Endoscopy and Gastroenterology Unit, Department of Pediatrics, "Santo Spirito" Hospital, Pescara, Italy
e-mail: mariateresa.illiceto@ausl.pe.it; giuliano.lombardi@ausl.pe.it

G. Lisi
Pediatric Surgery Unit, Department of Aging Science, University "G. d'Annunzio", Chieti-Pescara, Italy
e-mail: gabriele.lisi@unich.it

© Springer International Publishing AG, part of Springer Nature 2018
L. Dall'Oglio, C. Romano (eds.), *Endoscopy in Pediatric Inflammatory Bowel Disease*, https://doi.org/10.1007/978-3-319-61249-2_1

Table 1.1 Endoscope choice based on weight (ESGE-ESPGHAN guidelines)

Weight or age	EGD	Colonoscopy	ERCP
<10 kg or <1 year	≤6 mm gastroscope preferred. Consider standard adult gastroscope if endotherapy required	≤6 mm gastroscope, standard adult gastroscope or pediatric colonoscope.	7.5 mm duodenoscope
≥10 kg or >1 year	Standard adult gastroscope Therapeutic gastroscope if needed	Pediatric or adult colonoscope	Therapeutic duodenoscope (4.2 mm operative channel)

gastrointestinal tracts in even preterm newborns. Over the years several guidelines have been published, regarding the type of endoscopes to be used; we refer to the most recent ESGE-ESPGHAN guidelines (Table 1.1).

The three major manufacturers (Olympus, Fujinon, and Pentax) have pediatric product lines with similar characteristics. Each provides brilliant, high-resolution color views of the gastrointestinal mucosa through a wide angle. The depth of view ranges from 5 to 100 mm, with nearly a 30-fold magnification of the mucosa. Depending on the manufacturer, smaller-sized duodenoscopes, enteroscopes, and variable-stiffness colonoscopes can be found. In addition, adult operative (two-channel) gastroscopes and "zoom" gastroscopes allowing magnification (up to 150×) of the mucosal image have occasional applications in children.

In 2012, the American Society for Gastrointestinal Endoscopy (ASGE) Technology Committee drew up reviews of existing, new, or emerging endoscopic technologies that have an impact on the practice of gastrointestinal (GI) endoscopy [2]. More recently, in 2017, the European Society of Gastrointestinal Endoscopy (ESGE) and European Society for Paediatric Gastroenterology Hepatology and Nutrition (ESPGHAN) published the executive summary of the Guidelines on pediatric gastrointestinal endoscopy that refers to infants, children, and adolescents aged 0–18 years.

1.1.1 Esophagogastroduodenoscopy (EGD)

The choice of pediatric endoscope type is based on the age and weight of the patient, the presence of any anatomical anomalies, and the indication for the procedure (diagnostic and/or therapeutic) (Table 1.2) [2].

1.1.2 Neonatal Patients

Neonatal (ultrathin) gastroscopes are similar to standard gastroscopes in design and length, but some models have only two-way tip deflection (up/down) [3], and right/left view is obtained by rotating the shaft of the instrument. The smallest insertion tube diameter allows easy transit through the narrow pediatric lumens. Also the

Table 1.2 Neonatal (ultrathin) and pediatric gastroscopes (ASGE Technology Committee, 2012)

Manufacturer	Model	Insertion tube length/diameter, mm	Definition/magnification/ color enhancement	Biopsy channel/ diameter, mm
Olympus	GIF-N180	1100/4.9	Standard/none/NBI	1/2.0
	GIF-XP180N	1100/5.5	Standard/none/NBI	1/2.0
Fujinon	EG530N	1100/5.9	High-definition/zoom	1/2.0
	EG530NP	1100/4.9	High-definition/zoom	1/2.0
Pentax	EG1690K	1100/5.4	Standard/zoom/iSCAN	1/2.0
	EG1870K	1050/6.0	Standard/zoom/iSCAN	1/2.0

NBI narrow-band imaging

working channel of these endoscopes is narrower (1.5–2.0 mm), requiring the use of appropriate small-caliber accessories. Due to the small diameter of the working channel the suction capacity in case of bleeding is inadequate, so in these cases the use of a larger caliber endoscope is indicated.

1.1.3   Children Weighing less than 10–15 kg

In patients weighing less than 10–15 kg, gastroscopes with an outer diameter of 4.9–6.0 mm are preferred, particularly for those weighing less than 5 kg [4, 5]. In these patients, the use of larger diameter gastroscopes (both for diagnostic and therapeutic procedures) exhibits a high risk of mucosal damage, perforation, and tracheal compression.

1.1.4   Children Older than 12 Months or Weighing more than 10–15 kg

In most children older than 1 year and weighing more than 10–15 kg, gastroscopes with an outside diameter of 8 mm or larger may be used. However, most pediatric endoscopists start the examination with a smaller gastroscope, and eventually proceed with a larger caliber if the procedure requires it (bleeding, dilatation, …), compatibly with the ability of the instrument to pass beyond the physiological anatomic narrowings (upper esophageal sphincter, pylorus).

1.2   Colonoscopy

Pediatric colonoscopy is an instrumental test that is extremely useful in selected cases, but has specific peculiarities compared to adulthood, both for indications and for procedures.

The American Society for Gastrointestinal Endoscopy (ASGE) and the North American Society for Pediatric Gastroenterology Hepatology and Nutrition

Table 1.3 Typical diagnostic and therapeutic indications, non-indications, and contraindications for ileocolonoscopy in pediatric patients (ESGE-ESPGHAN 2017)

Diagnostic indications
  Unexplained anemia
  Unexplained chronic diarrhea
  Perianal lesions (fistula, abscess)
  Rectal blood loss
  Unexplained failure to thrive
  Suspicion of graft-versus-host disease
  Rejection or complications after intestinal transplantation Polyposis syndrome (diagnosis and surveillance)
  Radiological suspicion of ileocolonic stenosis/stricture
  Polyposis syndromes
Therapeutic indications
  Polypectomy
  Foreign-body removal
  Dilation of ileocolonic stenosis
  Treatment of hemorrhagic lesions
  Reduction of sigmoidal volvulus
Non-indications
  Functional GI disorders
  Constipation
Contraindications
  Toxic megacolon
  Recent colonic perforation
  Recent intestinal resection (<7 days)

(NASPGHAN) modified the previous guidelines, adding clear indications for pediatric endoscopy [6]. The ESGE-ESPGHAN guidelines revised the indications, both in terms of diagnosis and treatment (Table 1.3).

Pediatric colonoscopes have variable insertion tube lengths (1330–1700 mm), shaft diameters (9.8–11.8 mm), and channel size (2.8–3.8 mm) (Table 1.4).

There are no published data to support specific guidelines for a colonoscopes caliber in children, and recommendations are based on experience.

1.2.1   Neonatal Patients (<5 kg)

Children weighing less than 5 kg may undergo successful ileocolonoscopy with ultrathin gastroscopes, although the procedure may be difficult due to the flexibility of the insertion tube.

1.2.2   Children Weighing Between 5 and 12 kg

In children weighing between 5 and 12 kg, colonoscopy can be performed using a pediatric or adult standard gastroscope.

Table 1.4 Pediatric colonoscopies (ASGE Technology Committee, 2012)

Manufacturer	Model	Insertion tube length/diameter, mm	Definition/magnification/ color enhancement	Biopsy channel number/ diameter, mm
Olympus	PCF Q180 AL	1680/11.5	High resolution/none/NBI	1/3.2
	PCF Q180 AI	1330/11.5	High resolution/none/NBI	1/3.2
	PCF H180 AL	1680/11.8	High resolution/none/NBI	1/3.2
	PCF H180 AI	1330/11.8	High resolution/none/NBI	1/3.2
Fujinon	EC530 LS	1690/11.5	High-definition/zoom	1/3.8
	EC450 LS5	1690/11.5	High-definition/zoom	1/3.8
	EC450 LPS	1690/11.1	High-definition/zoom	1/3.2
Pentax	EC2990 Li	1700/9.8	High-definition/zoom/ iSCAN	1/2.8
	EC3490 Li	1700/11.6	High-definition/zoom/ iSCAN	1/3.2
	EC3490 LK	1700/11.6	High resolution/zoom/ iSCAN	1/3.8

NBI narrow-band imaging

1.2.3   Children Weighing more than 12–15 kg

A body weight of 12–15 kg represents the limit for the use of a standard pediatric colonoscopy [7].

The limitation of procedures carried out with a pediatric colonoscope with a 2.8-mm working channel is the impossibility to use larger accessories.

1.3   Capsule Endoscopy

Clinical use of the capsule endoscopy (CE) received the approval of the FDA in 2001, and it shortly became a modern approach in the exploration of the intestine, although, only recently, data on its application in pediatric gastroenterology are emerging [8]. In 2015, a review provides an up-to-date information about wireless capsule endoscopy in children, in the contest of a Journal Continuing-Medical-Education (CME) Activity by NASPGHAN [9].

Indications for CE in children provide evaluation of the small bowel mucosa in Crohn's disease, occult bleeding, polyposis, graft-versus-host disease, lymphangi-ectasia, growth failure, or abdominal pain [10–13].

This procedure is approved by the U.S. Food and Drug Administration for children 2 years old or older, but there are no guidelines on the lower age and weight limits (few cases are described of 8–10 months old infant in which the procedure was successfully performed) [14, 15].

The main problem for the procedure in children is their ability to swallow the capsule, which measures 11 × 26 mm. In patients who are either unable to swallow the capsule by age (below 4 years [13]), by refusal or fear (even in older children), or by anatomical abnormalities, the capsule can be placed directly in the stomach or duodenum with a trans-endoscopic delivery device of 2.5 mm in diameter, which requires the use of an endoscope working channel ≥2.8 mm.

CE has been performed safely in a small series of pediatric patients, always confirming its degree of safety and tolerability. In addition, several studies have reported greater sensitivity than radiological and standard endoscopic examination in the detection of small bowel Crohn's disease distribution, gastrointestinal bleeding source, and presence of polyps in children [16]. The limitation of capsule endoscopy is the inability to biopsy and treat small bowel lesions. Colon capsule endoscopy (CCE) is a minimally invasive technique specifically designed to explore the colon without sedation and air insufflation. This procedure has been assessed as a surrogate to colonoscopy in pediatric ulcerative colitis [17].

1.3.1 Small Bowel Enteroscopy

Endoscopic investigation of small bowel disorders in children has historically been difficult due to the length and tortuosity of the organ itself [18]. Factors influencing the choice of endoscope are similar to those listed for upper endoscopy. Performing an enteroscopy may be more difficult in children because of the smaller abdominal cavity.

1.3.2 Push Enteroscopy

Push enteroscopy can be performed using an enteroscope or pediatric colonoscope. Enteroscopes are available with an outer diameter of 8.5–11.6 mm, working lengths of 2000–2200 mm, and a channel size of 2.2–3.8 mm.

1.3.3 Antegrade and Retrograde Balloon-Assisted Enteroscopy

The introduction of balloon enteroscopy allows deep intubation of the small bowel, and at times viewing of the entire mucosal surface.

– *Double-Balloon enteroscopy* has been safely reported in children as small as 12 kg and youngest age 2 years, and has been successfully performed in children with Roux-en-Y anastomoses in the evaluation and therapy of biliary strictures. We must consider that procedures performed in children under 8–10 years of age present a greater risk of complications [19].

Double-balloon enteroscopes (Fujinon, Wayne, NJ) consist of a high-resolution video enteroscope (EN-450P5/20) with a flexible overtube (TS-12140), having working lengths of 1520–2000 mm, outer diameter of 8.5–9.4 mm, and channel size of 2.2–2.8 mm. The overtubes require measure 12.2–13.2 mm in outer diameter. The enteroscopes and overtube have balloons fitted at the distal tip of each, which are sequentially inflated and deflated with air from a pressure controlled pump system with a maximum inflatable pressure of 45 mmHg. Available devices include argon plasma coagulation probes, biopsy forceps, and polypectomy snares. Training and learning curves for this procedure are, it is estimated by the procedurists, similar to that encountered in ileocolonoscopy, and clearly it is not yet apparent in pediatric practice how many DBE procedures are necessary in order to attain a high degree of competence [20].

– *Single-balloon enteroscopy* has also been performed in pediatric children [21, 22], the smallest of which reported undergone an antegrade study was 3 years old and weighed 13.5 kg [23].

One single-balloon enteroscope system is available (Olympus Medical System) with a 9.2 mm outer diameter, a working length of 2000 mm and a 2.8-mm channel, with an overtube of 13.2 mm outer diameter.

Both procedures can be applied to patients who tolerate the diameter of the overtube.

1.4   Endoscopic Retrograde Cholangiopancreatography (ERCP)

The ERCP can be performed successfully and safely in children with complication rates comparable to those in adults. The type of cannulation and patient age are independent risk factors for complications [23].

The ESGE/ESPGHAN guidelines indicate ERCP in pediatric patients (>1 year old) for therapeutic purposes (chronic pancreatitis, recurrent acute pancreatitis, pancreas divisum, postsurgical/post-traumatic pancreatic duct leak, pancreatic pseudocyst, common bile duct stones, postsurgical/post-traumatic bile leak, benign and/or malignant biliary strictures, primary sclerosing cholangitis often associated with inflammatory bowel disease, parasitosis) following diagnostic information from noninvasive modalities, while diagnostic ERCP can be considered in selected cases (evaluation of anomalous biliopancreatic junction, cholestasis in neonates and infants, choledochal cyst, and primary sclerosing cholangitis), performing the procedure with a pediatric 7.5-mm duodenoscope (2-mm working channel) in children weighing <10 kg, using a therapeutic duodenoscope (10.8–12.1 mm outer diameter) in those weighing ≥10 kg (although the soft-walled trachea in young children may become compressed because of the large diameter) [24, 25].

1.4.1   Endoscopic Ultrasonography (EUS)

The application of endoscopic ultrasound (EUS) in children is growing, with studies demonstrating a positive impact of EUS in the management of childhood diseases.

EUS has shown to be useful in the evaluation and management of a spectrum of childhood diseases including pancreaticobiliary disease, congenital anomalies, submucosal lesions, biliary stones disease, inflammatory bowel disease, and eosinophilic esophagitis. Its diagnostic capabilities with fine-needle aspiration and core-needle biopsy are shown to be technically successful, safe, and effective in several pediatric studies. Therapeutic EUS procedures include endoscopic cystgastrostomy, celiac plexus neurolysis, and biliary access [26–28]. There are no specific equipment for children. Standard radial echoendoscopes have a tip diameter ranging from 12.7 to 14.2 mm, and linear FNA echoendoscopes are slightly larger, measuring 12.1–14.6 mm in tip diameter.

In children weighing >15 kg a standard echo-endoscope should be employed only under general anesthesia, considering the stiff and potentially traumatic rigid distal part, requiring strict collaboration between adult and pediatric gastroenterologists [25].

The endobronchial ultrasound (EBUS) endoscope can be adapted for EUS in children with a weight below 15 kg.

Through-the-scope miniprobes with frequencies ranging from 12 to 30 MHz may be used through a 2.8-mm working channel of a standard gastroscope, in infant as young as 5 months of age. In smaller infants, a 1.7-mm miniprobe is available.

1.4.2   Biopsy Forceps

Mucosal biopsies are an essential component of most pediatric endoscopic procedures. Forceps available for 2-mm channel have fenestrated and serrated designs, with and without a needle-spike and with oval or alligator-type cups.

Large-cup forceps have been used in children without complications, but the utility of a larger tissue specimen is uncertain in pediatric population.

1.4.3   Endoscopic Retrieval Devices

To remove foreign bodies, there are several devices compatible with 2-mm working channels, such as retrieval snares, retrieval nets, alligator jaw, rat-tooth, and 3-prong graspers, as well as baskets [29]. There are no published data on the use of overtubes in children, because it is rarely used due to the high risk of injury to the esophagus or pharynx.

1.4.4   Polypectomy Devices

Most children requiring a polypectomy have an age and weight that allows using probes with a 2.8-mm working channel, but there are also polypectomy snares for use through a 2.0-mm channel.

1.4.5 Hemostatic Devices

Pediatric hemostasis techniques do not differ from those of the adult, and include: injection therapy, mechanical closure, and thermal techniques (multipolar/bipolar electrocautery, heater probe, and argon plasma coagulation).

In the last few years, hemostatic powders have been introduced for the endoscopic management of hemorrhagic lesions, either venous or arterial, and treatment of bleeding from malignant masses in adult patients [30–34].

1.4.6 Devices for Esophageal and Ileocolonic Dilation

Dilation of esophageal strictures in pediatric patients has been performed for decades [35]. Endoscopic dilators and techniques have been reported and depend on the stricture's etiology, the availability of different tools, and the operator's experience and preferences (Fig. 1.1).

At the beginning, the only dilators available were the Maloney dilators, which were passed under guidance of the rigid esophagoscope or blindly.

As soon as balloons and the Savary-Gilliard (S-G) dilators became available, blind bougienage was abandoned [36].

Balloon and semirigid dilators are the most frequently used tools. No high-quality studies have reported on the differences in the efficacies and rates of complications associated with these two types of dilators.

In patients with Crohn's disease (CD), strictures typically are found in terminal ileum and colon as well as the site of ileocolonic surgical anastomosis. Endoscopic balloon dilation in patients with symptomatic CD strictures of the small bowel has a durable clinical response. Two retrospective series found technical success rates of 89–97%, and serious adverse events were reported in 5%. Dilating balloons >20 mm appear to be associated with more adverse events [37].

1.4.6.1 Bougie Dilators
Bougie dilators can be passed across esophageal strictures by applying axial and radial force to the narrowed region.

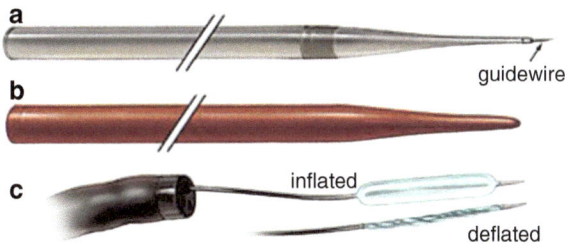

Fig. 1.1 Esophageal dilators: (**a**) Savary, (**b**) Maloney, (**c**) Through-the-scope (TTS) balloon catheter

- Available bougie dilators include Savary-Gilliard (Cook Endoscopy), which are tapered with a radiopaque marker at the base of the taper. These polyvinyl wire-guided dilators have various diameters (5–20 mm or 15F–60F) and lengths (70 or 100 cm). They are safer and more effective than balloon dilators in the treatment of consolidated and old cicatricial strictures and in cases of resistant esophageal narrowing due to, e.g., congenital esophageal stenosis (CES) with cartilaginous remnants [38].
- American Dilation System dilators are similar but have a shorter taper tip and are radiopaque throughout their length.
- Tucker dilators are especially useful in the treatment of tortuous strictures secondary to caustic ingestions [39]. These are small silicone bougies, tapered at each end with loops that can be pulled antegrade or retrograde across very tight strictures regardless of length. A gastrostomy is required for use. In very tight strictures where there is the possibility of complete lumen occlusion, a string must be maintained across the stricture emerging from both the nose and gastrostomy site between dilations. Tucker dilators range in size from 4 to 13.3 mm (12F–40F).

1.4.6.2 Through-the-Scope Balloon

Balloon dilation can be performed in infants who will not tolerate a standard gastroscope by using a guidewire and over-the-wire dilation balloons (e.g., biliary dilation balloons) under fluoroscopic guidance. Biliary dilation balloons are available in sizes ranging from 4 to 10 mm with lengths from 2 to 8 cm and can be used with endoscopically placed 0.035-inch guidewires. The advantages of balloon dilators include the radial force that is applied to the stenosis and the avoidance of the application of axial force. Balloon dilators can be advanced through the endoscope channel and carefully pushed forward into and through the stenosis under direct vision. Balloon dilators may also be inserted, on the side of the endoscope itself or under fluoroscopic control, over a guidewire that has previously been inserted through the scope [40].

Pneumatic dilation for treatment of achalasia in children is successfully performed [41].

1.4.6.3 Esophageal Stents

There are no esophageal stents designed for pediatric use.

Two different strategies for stenting have been described.

- Rigid stent: the metal and plastic stents press against the esophageal wall, with food and secretions that pass through the stent itself.
- Dynamic stent: a plastic or silicon tube fixed to a nasogastric tube. Food and secretions passing repeatedly in the space between the stenosis and the stent itself seem to effectively maintaining lumen patency [42].

The use of plastic and nitinol esophageal and airway stents has been reported in treating recalcitrant esophageal strictures in children in case series [43]. The smaller diameter (10–20 mm) and shorter length (20–80 mm) of the airway stents may make them more suitable in smaller patients [43, 44], such as endoscopic biliary accessories safely used to dilate refractory esophageal strictures [45].

The choice of a particular stent must be based on the location and characteristics of the stricture as well as the size of the patient.

1.5   Conclusion and Future Directions

Pediatric gastrointestinal endoscopy continues to evolve favorably, and provides a safe and effective diagnostic tool. The most frequently performed procedures are EGD and colonoscopy. Wireless capsule endoscopy or double-balloon enteroscopy for investigation of the small intestine can be performed alternatively to magnetic resonance enteroclysis, which remains the only choice in infants. Therapeutic procedures such as polypectomy, endoscopic hemostasis of gastrointestinal bleeding, retrieval of foreign bodies, ERCP, or ligation of esophageal varices can also be performed in infants.

Endoscopy is fundamental to the care of IBD: It is used to make an initial diagnosis, distinguish CD from ulcerative colitis, assess disease extent and activity, monitor response to therapy, survey for dysplasia, and provide endoscopic treatment such as ileocolonic dilation. A further application in pediatric IBD concerns the ileal pouch endoscopy in patients with ulcerative colitis (UC) who require colectomy (for the endoscopic and histological assessment of pouchitis, pouch leakage, or other local disease), and colorectal cancer screening and surveillance, in patients with long-standing UC and extensive CD colitis who are at risk for development of dysplasia and colorectal cancer [37].

In recent years, the increased use of pediatric endoscopy in clinical practice is stimulating industry to produce specific tools and accessories, although a greater availability of pediatric instruments and accessories would be desirable.

References

1. Fox VL. Pediatric endoscopy. In: Classen M, Tytgat GNJ, Lightdale CJ, editors. Gastroenterology endoscopy. Stuttgart, Germany/New York: Thieme; 2002. p. 720–52.
2. ASGE Technology Committee. Status evaluation report equipment for pediatric endoscopy. Gastrointest Endosc. 2012;76(1):8–17.
3. Rodriguez SA, Banerjee S, Desilets D, et al. Ultrathin endoscopes. Gastrointest Endosc. 2010;71:893–8.
4. Benaroch LM, Rudolph CD. Introduction to pediatric esophagogastroduodenoscopy and enteroscopy. Gastrointest Endosc. 2010;71:893–8.
5. Schappi MGMJ, Mougenot J-F, Belli DC, et al. Upper gastrointestinal endoscopy. In: Kleinman R, Olivier G, Miele-Vergani G, et al., editors. Walker's pediatric gastrointestinal disease: physiology, diagnosis, management, vol. 2. 5th ed. Decker: Hamilton, ON, Canada; 2008. p. 1265–83.
6. North American Society for Pediatric Gastroenterology, Hepatology and Nutrition; and American Society for Gastrointestinal Endoscopy. Modifications in endoscopic practice for pediatric patients. Gastrointest Endosc. 2008;67:1–9.

7. Thomson M. Colonoscopy and enteroscopy. Gastrointest Endosc Clin N Am. 2001;11:603–39, vi.
8. de'Angelis GL, Fornaroli F, et al. Wireless capsule endoscopy for pediatric small-bowel diseases. Am J Gastroenter. 2007;102:1749–57.
9. Zevit N, Shamir R. Wireless capsule endoscopy of the small intestine in children. J Pediatr Gastroenterol Nutr. 2015;60:696–701.
10. Seidman EG, Sant'Anna AM, Dirks MH. Potential applications of wireless capsule endoscopy in the pediatric age group. Gastrointest Endosc Clin N Am. 2004;14:207–17.
11. Guilhon de Araujo Sant'Anna AM, Dubois J, Miron MC, et al. Wireless capsule endoscopy for obscure small-bowel disorders: final results of the first pediatric controlled trial. Clin Gastroenterol Hepatol. 2005;3:264–70.
12. Antao B, Bishop J, Shawis R, et al. Clinical application and diagnostic yield of wireless capsule endoscopy in children. J Laparoendosc Adv Surg Tech A. 2007;17:364–70.
13. Fritscher-Ravens A, Scherbakov P, Bufler P, et al. The feasibility of wireless capsule endoscopy in detecting small intestinal pathology in children under the age of 8 years: a multicenter European study. Gut. 2009;58:1467–72.
14. Nuutinen H, Kolho KL, Salminem P, Rintala R, et al. Capsule endoscopy in pediatric patients: technique and results in our first 100 consecutive children. Scandin J Gastroenterol. 2011;46(9):1138–43.
15. Jensen MK, Tipnis NA, Bajorunaite R, et al. Capsule endoscopy performed across the pediatric age range: indications, incomplete studies and utility in management of inflammatory bowel disease. Gastrointest Endosc. 2010;72:95–102.
16. Thomson M, Fritscher-Ravens A, Mylonaki M, Swain P, et al. Wireless capsule endoscopy in children: a study to assess diagnostic yield in small bowel disease in paediatric patients. J Ped Gastroenterol Nutr. 2007;44(2):192–7.
17. Spada X, Hasan C, et al. Colon capsule endoscopy: European Society of Gastrointestinal Endoscopy (ESGE) guideline. Endoscopy. 2012;44(5):527–36.
18. Barth BA. Enteroscopy in children. Curr Opin Pediatr. 2011;23(5):530–4.
19. Yokohama K, Yano T, Kumagai H, et al. Double-balloon enteroscopy for pediatric patients: evaluation of safety and efficacy in 257 cases. J Pediatr Gastroenterol Nutr. 2016;63(1):34–40.
20. Thomson M, Venkatesh K, et al. Double balloon enteroscopy in children: diagnosis, treatment and safety. World J Gastroenterol. 2010;16(1):56–62.
21. Barth BA, Channabasappa N. Single-balloon enteroscopy in children: initial experience at a pediatric center. J Pediatr Gastroenterol Nutr. 2010;51:680–4.
22. Oliva S, Pennazio M, et al. Capsule endoscopy followed by single balloon enteroscopy in children with obscure gastrointestinal bleeding: a combined approach. Dig Liver Dis. 2015;47(2):125–30.
23. Kramer RE, Brumbaugh DE, Soden JS, et al. First successful antegrade single-balloon enteroscopy in a 3-year-old with occult GI bleeding. Gastrointest Endosc. 2009;70:546–9.
24. Rosen JD, Lane RS, Mrtinez JM, et al. Success and safety of endoscopic retrograde cholangiopancreatography in children. J Pediatr Surg. 2017;52(7):1148–51.
25. Tringali A, Thomson M, et al. Pediatric gastrointestinal endoscopy: European Society of Gastrointestinal Endoscopy (ESGE) and European Society for Paediatric Gastroenterology Hepatology and Nutrition (ESPGHAN) guideline executive summary. Endoscopy. 2017;49(1):83–91.
26. Patel S, Marshak J, et al. The emerging role of endoscopic ultrasound for pancreaticobiliary diseases in the pediatric population. World J Pediatr. 2017;13(4):300–6. https://doi.org/10.1007/s12519-017-0020-y.
27. Mahajan R, Simon EG, et al. Endoscopic ultrasonography in pediatric patients—experience from a tertiary care center in India. Indian J Gastroenterol. 2016;35(1):14–9.
28. Lakhole A, Liu QY. Role of endoscopic ultrasound in pediatric disease. Gastrointest Endosc Clin N Am. 2016;26(1):137–53.
29. Diehl DL, Adler DG, et al. Endoscopic retrieval devices. Gastrointest Endosc. 2009;69:997–1003.

30. McKiernan PJ, Beath SV, Davison SM, et al. A prospective study of endoscopic esophageal variceal ligation using a multiband ligator. J Pediatr Gastroenterol Nutr. 2002;34:207–11.
31. Gershman G, Thomson M. Therapeutic upper GI endoscopy. In: Practical pediatric gastrointestinal endoscopy. 2nd ed. Oxford, UK: Wiley-Blackwell. p. 82–92.
32. Paganelli M, Alvarez F, et al. Use of hemospray for non-variceal esophageal bleeding in an infant. J Hepatol. 2014;61(3):712–3.
33. Prei JC, Barmeyer C, et al. EndoClot Polysaccharide Hemostatic System in nonvariceal gastrointestinal bleeding: results of a prospective multicenter observational pilot study. J Clin Gastroenterol. 2016;50(10):e98–e100.
34. Bustamante-Balén M, Plumé G. Role of hemostatic powders in the endoscopic management of gastrointestinal bleeding. World J Gastrointest Pathophysiol. 2014;5(3):284–92.
35. Antoniou D, Soutis M, Christopoulos-Geroulanos G. Anastomotic strictures following esophageal atresia repair: a 20-year experience with endoscopic balloon dilatation. J Pediatr Gastroenterol Nutr. 2010;51:464–7.
36. Christopoulos-Geroulanos G. Experience with esophageal dilatations in children. Ann Gastroenterol. 2003;16(2):151–4.
37. ASGE Standard of Practice Committee. Guideline: the role of endoscopy in inflammatory bowel disease. Gastrointest Endosc. 2015;81(5):1101–21.
38. Romeo E, Foschia F, de Angelis P, et al. Endoscopic management of congenital esophageal stenosis. J Pediatr Surg. 2011;46(5):838–41.
39. Saleem MM. Acquired oesophageal strictures in children: emphasis on the use of string-guided dilatations. Singap Med J. 2009;50:82–6.
40. Dall'Oglio L, Caldaro T, Foschia F, et al. Endoscopic management of esophageal stenosis in children: new and traditional treatments. World J Gastrointest Endosc. 2016;8(4):212–9.
41. Pastor AC, Mills J, Marcon MA, et al. A single center 26-year experience with treatment of esophageal achalasia: is there an optimal method? J Pediatr Surg. 2009;44:1349–54.
42. Caldaro T, Torroni F, De Angelis P, et al. Dynamic esophageal stents. Dis Esophagus. 2013;26:388–91.
43. Best C, Sudel B, Foker JE, et al. Esophageal stenting in children: indications, application, effectiveness and complications. Gastrointest Endosc. 2009;70:1248–53.
44. Broto J, Asensio M, Vernet JM. Results of a new technique in the treatment of severe esophageal stenosis in children: poliflex stents. J Pediatr Gastroenterol Nutr. 2003;37:203–6.
45. Gebrail R, Absah I. Successful use of esophageal stent placement to treat a postoperative esophageal stricture in a toddler. ACG Case Rep J. 2014;2(1):61–3.

Bowel Preparation and Factors Correlated with Patients and Parents

2

Claudio Romano and Valeria Dipasquale

2.1 Introduction

Colonoscopy is the current standard procedure performed in children to investigate various gastrointestinal conditions. The diagnostic and therapeutic efficacy of colonoscopy greatly depends on the quality of the colonic cleansing or preparation [1]. Other procedures that require colonic preparation are video capsule endoscopy and, more recently, double-balloon enteroscopy. Colonic cleansing for colonoscopy in children should prioritize safety and palatability and take into consideration patient's age, clinics, and compliance [2]. To date, no identified standard practice exists, and pediatric colonic cleansing regimens vary greatly among medical centers and individual healthcare providers.

2.2 Bowel Preparation

2.2.1 Bowel Cleansing Solutions

The ideal solution for colonoscopy would clear the colon of all fecal material with neither macroscopic nor microscopic alteration of the colonic mucosa; moreover, it would avoid patient discomfort or fluid and electrolyte shifts and would also be safe, tolerable, and inexpensive [3]. At present, various bowel cleansing solutions are available for pediatric patients, but none of them present all these characteristics. Laxatives are substances that stimulate defecation and soften hardened feces, impacting on the transfer of fluid and electrolytes in the small and large intestine.

C. Romano (✉) · V. Dipasquale
Pediatric Gastroenterology and Cystic Fibrosis Unit, Department of Human Pathology in Adulthood and Childhood "G. Barresi", University of Messina, Messina, Italy
e-mail: romanoc@unime.it

Laxatives are usually administered orally for bowel preparation and, according to their mode of action, are divided into stimulant and osmotic [3, 4].

Stimulant laxatives are represented by bisacodyl and senna. They have secretory and prokinetic mechanisms of action and are usually administered at low dosages, in association with other laxatives. Reported cleaning power is good, up to 92–93% of cases along with other laxatives [5], especially polyethylene glycol-3350 (PEG-3350), a specific PEG product. Nonetheless, they are poorly tolerable because of colicky abdominal pain and/or electrolytes disturbances, especially if used in monotherapy at higher doses.

Osmotic laxatives that have been used in bowel preparation include magnesium citrate, sodium phosphate, PEG-3350, and PEG with electrolytes (PEG-ELS) [3]. Magnesium citrate and sodium phosphate are hyperosmotic laxatives. They act osmotically by determining the intraluminal fluid and electrolytes accumulation, but also have a prokinetic mechanism of action by stimulating the action of cholecystokinin (CCK). Magnesium citrate alone or in combination with a stimulant or PEG seems to be effective, but tolerance varies in the pediatric population. Use with caution is recommended in renal failure, since magnesium is excreted via the kidneys. Sodium phosphate preparations use (oral or enema) is forbidden in patients younger than age 18 years, because it can cause acute phosphate nephropathy with acute and/or chronic tubular injury [6]. Hyperosmotic laxatives use is discouraged in critical ill patient and inflammatory bowel disease (IBD) patient, since they carry high risk of electrolytes disturbances. They can also alter colonic mucosa, resulting in false mucosal injuries.

PEG-based solutions are isosmotic, nonabsorbable solutions, designed to pass through the bowel without neither absorption nor secretion, with clinically insignificant electrolyte changes and less discomfort for the patient. Currently, different PEG-based formulations are available. PEG-3350 has good tolerance and effective cleansing power in up to 93% of cases [7]; it is recommended the combination with electrolyte solutions to prevent electrolyte imbalance, since isosmotic preparations that contain PEG are osmotically balanced with nonfermentable electrolyte solutions. The use of PEG-ELS is one of the most common methods of cleansing the colon in children [2]; it is safe in case of pre-existing electrolyte imbalances and does not alter the histologic features of the colonic mucosa. For all these reasons it may be safely used in patients with renal failure, congestive heart failure, and suspected IBD [4]. Despite a good safety profile, 5–15% of patients do not complete the preparation because of poor tolerance: responsible characteristics are the unpleasant sulfate-associated taste and the large volume of fluids required (4 L have traditionally been used to achieve a cathartic effect) [8], which can cause abdominal fullness and cramping. PEG-ELS gut lavage via nasogastric (NG) tube is the most effective method for colonic cleansing in infants and children. PEG-ELS is not approved for children younger than 6 months [3].

Prepopik is another osmotic agent approved in 2012 in adults. It had been available and in use only in Canada, sold as Pico-Salax. Some studies have demonstrated a good efficacy and tolerance profile in children too, also in comparison to PEG-ELS [9, 10].

Table 2.1 Clear liquids guidelines [3]	Clear liquids suggested	Water
		Jell-O
		Soda
		Ice
		Popsicles
		Clear broth
		Pedialyte
		Clear juice drinks without pulp
		Sports drink
	Avoid	Red liquids
		Solid foods
		Milk or milk products
		Juice with pulp

2.2.2   Bowel Cleanout Regimens

Uniform standard protocols have not been generally accepted despite the thousands of pediatric colonoscopies performed worldwide. Each gastroenterology program generally elaborates its own unique protocol, which may differ from others. The North American Society for Pediatric Gastroenterology, Hepatology, and Nutrition (NASPGHAN) Endoscopy and Procedures Committee, and the American Society for Gastrointestinal Endoscopy (ASGE) Standards of Practice Committee reviewed the literature data and evidence and suggested best practice recommendations [3, 4]. For infants younger than 2 years of age, ingestion of clear liquids for 24 h prior to the examination and a normal saline solution enema (5 mL/kg) would be sufficient [4, 11]. Recommended and forbidden liquids for bowel preparation are listed in Table 2.1. For children older than 2 years of age, cleansing can be accomplished with intestinal cleanout by using osmotic agents, such as PEG-based solutions with and without electrolytes, dietary restrictions, stimulant laxatives, and/or enemas [3, 4]. PEG-ELS has to be used as the primary agent for bowel cleansing [2]. Administration via a NG tube in a hospital setting for 24 h before the procedure is a safe and appropriate regimen, especially in children younger than 6 years of age [4, 11]. There is a wide range of PEG-based preparation regimens (Table 2.2). Several studies have reported on the safety and efficacy of 4-day bowel preparations by using PEG-3350 without electrolytes in children [12, 13]. Other studies have concluded that both 2-day [5, 14, 15] and 1-day [7, 16, 17] preparations are safe and effective. Low-volume PEG-ELS preparations have been formulated to provide a more tolerable bowel preparation. To date, low-volume 2-L PEG-ELS with ascorbic acid is the only FDA-approved low-volume PEG-ELS preparation commercially available. Adult studies have demonstrated an efficacy profile as good as that of 4-L-PEG-ELS [18]. Pediatric data are lacking.

Low-fiber diet for more than 24 h prior to the examination is not recommended in adults. Similarly, the routine use of enemas and prokinetic agents (such as metoclopramide, domperidone) is not recommended to be added to oral bowel preparation. Simethicone addition is suggested in order to ameliorate visualization of the mucosa. Data on children are not yet available [19].

Table 2.2 Common PEG-based preparation regimens [4]

Protocol	Dose and administration	Diet	Enema	Comments
PEG-ELS (short protocol)	100 mL/year of age/h for 4 h or 20 mL/kg/h (max rate of 1 L/h) for 4 h	Liberal until cleansing initiated (such as the afternoon before), then clears only until procedure	Only if no clear evacuations are obtained up to 1 h before procedure	Poor palatability and difficult to tolerate in most children; NG tube administration should be performed if requested volume has not been assumed after 1 h
PEG-ELS (long protocol)	100 mL/year of age/h over 24 h or 20 mL/kg/h (max rate of 1 L/h) over 24 h	Liberal until cleansing initiated, then clears only until procedure	Only if no clear evacuations are obtained up to 1 h before procedure	No pediatric trials
PEG-3350 (long protocol)	1.5 g/kg/day (max dose: 100 g/day) over 4 day mixed in a sports drink	Liberal until day before procedure, final 24 h should be clear fluids	On the day before procedure	No pediatric trials
PEG-3350 (short protocol)	238 g OTC (255-g prescription) in 1.9 L of a sports drink over 2–4 h on the day before procedure	Liberal until prep initiated, then clear liquids only	On the day before procedure	No pediatric trials

2.3 Bowel Preparation Quality

2.3.1 Documentation of Preparation Quality

Preparation quality has to be properly documented in colonoscopy reports. According to the U.S. Multi-Society Task Force on Colorectal Cancer, an examination is adequate when lesions other than small (5 mm) polyps are not obscured by residual colonic materials [20]. In clinical practice, preparation quality should be graded after efforts to remove residual effluent and fecal debris have been completed. Various validated scoring systems have been designed to rate the quality of colonoscopy preparation in clinical trials; no validated pediatric colon cleanliness index exists yet [2]. The Boston Bowel Preparation Score is currently the most used and standardized, both valid and reliable [21]. It uses a 10-point (0–9) summation score assessing bowel preparation quality in three segments of the colon after all cleansing procedures during colonoscopy have been completed (Table 2.3).

2.3.2 Inadequate Bowel Preparation

An effective bowel preparation represents a fundamental requirement for the success of colonoscopy. It allows: clear visualization of the colonic mucosa; detection of even minor injuries; complete procedures, up to terminal ileum (for colonoscopy)

Table 2.3 The Boston Bowel Preparation Scale [21]

Boston Bowel Preparation Scale rating for each colon segment	0	Unprepared colon segment with stool that cannot be cleared
	1	Portion of mucosa in segment seen after cleaning, but other areas not seen because of retained material
	2	Minor residual material after cleaning, but mucosa of segment generally well seen
	3	Entire mucosa of segment well seen after cleaning

Total score is calculated by adding the scores of the right, transverse, and left colon segments. The total Boston Bowel Preparation Scale score ranges from 0 (very poor) to 9 (excellent).

and caecum (with video capsule endoscopy); safe therapeutic procedures (such as polypectomy, hemostatic therapy, balloon dilation, and placement of percutaneous endoscopic gastrostomy tubes). On the contrary, suboptimal colonoscopy exposes to the risk of missed diagnosis, increased procedural time and risks, and increased costs from repeated procedures. Suboptimal colonic preparation can occur in up to one-third of colonoscopies [3]. In adult population, the most important predictor of inadequate preparation is a previous inadequate preparation. Other independent factors that have been shown to predict poor colon preparation include later colonoscopy starting time, failure to follow preparation instructions, hospitalized patients, procedural indication of constipation, use of tricyclic antidepressants, male sex, and a history of cirrhosis, stroke, or dementia. Obesity may also be a predictor of inadequate colon preparation [22, 23]. There is no standardized approach to an inadequately prepared colon discovered on intubation, and pediatric studies lack. Several irrigation devices have been developed to allow more aggressive water instillation, compared with standard irrigation pumps or syringe-based flushing [24]. In adults, it is recommended to offer a repeat colonoscopy within 1 year [22].

2.4   Parents' Preparation

In childhood, preparation for endoscopy requires attention to physiologic issues as well as the emotional and psychosocial well-being of both patients and parents. As with adults, anxiety about endoscopic procedures is frequent, because of the requirement of sedation or general anesthesia for pain, the potential for rare procedural accidents such as bleeding or intestinal perforation, and discomfort associated with the examination itself. Pain experience seems to be the most common concern of pediatric patients, while the risk of procedural accidents related to the endoscopy is parents' one [25]. A preparatory intervention could be useful to reduce anxiety experienced by both pediatric patients and parents. It has to include a thorough explanation regarding specific concerns.

Conclusion

An effective bowel preparation is crucial to increase the success rate of colonoscopy. PEG-ELS-based preparation is the primary agent for bowel cleansing, with both good efficacy and safety profiles. Large volume of fluids (4 L) is required to achieve a cathartic effect, so that administration via a nasogastric tube is often required in children. Low-volume 2-L PEG-ELS seems to have similar efficacy profile, but further pediatric data are warranted. The Boston Bowel Preparation Score is currently the most used index to rate the quality of bowel preparation before colonoscopy.

References

1. Rex DK, Petrini JL, Baron TH, et al. ASGE/ACG Taskforce on Quality in Endoscopy. Quality indicators for colonoscopy. Am J Gastroenterol. 2006;101:873–85.
2. Hunter A, Mamula P. Bowel preparation for pediatric colonoscopy procedures. J Pediatr Gastroenterol Nutr. 2010;51:254–61.
3. Pall H, Zacur GM, Kramer RE, et al. Bowel preparation for pediatric colonoscopy: report of the NASPGHAN Endoscopy and Procedures Committee. J Pediatr Gastroenterol Nutr. 2014;59:409–16.
4. ASGE Standards of Practice Committee, Lightdale JR, Acosta R, Shergill AK, et al. Modifications in endoscopic practice for pediatric patients. Gastrointest Endosc. 2014;79:699–710.
5. Phatak UP, Johnson S, Husain SZ, et al. Two-day bowel preparation with polyethylene glycol 3350 and bisacodyl: a new, safe, and effective regimen for colonoscopy in children. J Pediatr Gastroenterol Nutr. 2011;53:71–4.
6. US Food and Drug Administration. Information for healthcare professionals: oral sodium phosphate (OSP) products for bowel cleansing (marketed as Visicol and OsmoPrep, and oral sodium phosphate products available without a prescription). 2008. http://www.fda.gov/drugs/drugsafety/postmarketdrugsafetyinformationforpatientsandproviders/ucm126084.htm. Accessed 1 May 2014.
7. Adamiak T, Altaf M, Jensen MK, et al. One-day bowel preparation with polyethylene glycol 3350: an effective regimen for colonoscopy in children. Gastrointest Endosc. 2010;71:573–7.
8. Marshall JB, Pineda JJ, Barthel JS, et al. Prospective, randomized trial comparing sodium phosphate solution with polyethylene glycol electrolyte lavage for colonoscopy preparation. Gastrointest Endosc. 1993;39:631–4.
9. Jimenez-Rivera C, Haas D, Boland M, et al. Comparison of two common outpatient preparations for colonoscopy in children and youth. Gastroenterol Res Pract. 2009;2009:518932.
10. Turner D, Benchimol EI, Dunn H, et al. Pico-Salax versus polyethylene glycol for bowel cleanout before colonoscopy in children: a randomized controlled trial. Endoscopy. 2009;41:1038–45.
11. Turner D, Levine A, Weiss B, et al. Evidence-based recommendations for bowel cleansing before colonoscopy in children: a report from a national working group. Endoscopy. 2010;42:1063–70.
12. Pashankar DS, Uc A, Bishop WP. Polyethylene glycol 3350 without electrolytes: a new safe, effective, and palatable bowel preparation for colonoscopy in children. J Pediatr. 2004;144:358–62.
13. Safder S, Demintieva Y, Rewalt M, et al. Stool consistency and stool frequency are excellent clinical markers for adequate colon preparation after polyethylene glycol 3350 cleansing protocol: a prospective clinical study in children. Gastrointest Endosc. 2008;68:1131–5.
14. Jibaly R, LaChance J, Lecea NA, et al. The utility of PEG3350 without electrolytes for 2-day colonoscopy preparation in children. Eur J Pediatr Surg. 2011;21:318–21.
15. Terry NA, Chen-Lim ML, Ely E, et al. Polyethylene glycol powder solution vs. senna for bowel preparation for colonoscopy in children: a prospective, randomized, investigator-blinded trial. J Pediatr Gastroenterol Nutr. 2013;56:215–9.
16. Abbas MI, Nylund CM, Bruch CJ, et al. Prospective evaluation of 1-day polyethylene glycol-3350 bowel preparation regimen in children. J Pediatr Gastroenterol Nutr. 2013;56:220–4.

17. Najafi M, Fallahi GH, Motamed F, et al. Comparison of one and two-day bowel preparation with polyethylene glycol in pediatric colonoscopy. Turk J Gastroenterol. 2015;26:232–5.
18. Valiante F, Pontone S, Hassan C, et al. A randomized controlled trial evaluating a new 2-L PEG solution plus ascorbic acid vs 4-L PEG for bowel cleansing prior to colonoscopy. Dig Liver Dis. 2012;44:224–7.
19. Hassan C, Bretthauer M, Kaminski MF, et al. Bowel preparation for colonoscopy: European Society of Gastrointestinal Endoscopy (ESGE) guideline. Endoscopy. 2013;45:142–50.
20. Rex DK, Bond JH, Winawer S, et al. Quality in the technical performance of colonoscopy and the continuous quality improvement process for colonoscopy: recommendations of the U.S. Multi-Society Task Force on Colorectal Cancer. Am J Gastroenterol. 2002;97:1296–308.
21. Calderwood AH, Jacobson BC. Comprehensive validation of the Boston Bowel Preparation Scale. Gastrointest Endosc. 2010;72:686–92.
22. ASGE Standards of Practice Committee, Saltzman JR, Cash BD, Pasha SF, et al. Bowel preparation before colonoscopy. Gastrointest Endosc. 2015;81:781–94.
23. Fayad NF, Kahi CJ, Abd El-Jawad KH, et al. Association between body mass index and quality of split bowel preparation. Clin Gastroenterol Hepatol. 2013;11:1478–85.
24. Rigaux J, Juriens I, Devière J. A novel system for the improvement of colonic cleansing during colonoscopy. Endoscopy. 2012;44:703–6.
25. Hagiwara S, Nakayama Y, Tagawa M, et al. Pediatric patient and parental anxiety and impressions related to initial gastrointestinal endoscopy: a Japanese multicenter questionnaire study. Scientifica (Cairo). 2015;2015:797564.

Sedation

3

Claudio Romano and Valeria Dipasquale

3.1 Introduction

Gastrointestinal endoscopic procedures are fundamental to the assessment and treatment of a variety of gastrointestinal diseases. In pediatrics, anesthesia or deep sedation is almost always necessary to ensure patient safety, comfort, and cooperation [1]. Effective and safe sedation for pediatric endoscopic procedures is a non-negotiable pre-requisite. It mostly depends on the professional skills of the medical and nursing team, the appropriate selection and preparation of the patient, and the adequate management of pain by the use of analgesia.

3.2 Anesthesiologists Versus Non-anesthesiologists

General anesthesia by a multidisciplinary team led by an anesthesiologist is preferred. General anesthesia is possible not in all centers because of the limited availability of anesthesiologists. In many European countries and in parts of the United States, anesthesia departments cannot cope with the rising demands [2], and most pediatric gastroenterologists are well trained and certified to provide moderate sedation without anesthetic teams, in conformity with national and institutional regulations. Almost all gastrointestinal endoscopic procedures are performed while using either endoscopist-administered moderate sedation or anesthesiologist-administered deep sedation and general anesthesia [1, 3].

The choice depends on many patient- and procedure-related factors. Of great importance is the physical status assessment as codified by the American Society of Anesthesiology (ASA) (Table 3.1) [4]. If the child fits to ASA class I or II, sedation

C. Romano (✉) · V. Dipasquale
Pediatric Gastroenterology and Cystic Fibrosis Unit, Department of Human Pathology in Adulthood and Childhood "G. Barresi", University of Messina, Messina, Italy
e-mail: romanoc@unime.it

© Springer International Publishing AG, part of Springer Nature 2018
L. Dall'Oglio, C. Romano (eds.), *Endoscopy in Pediatric Inflammatory Bowel Disease*,
https://doi.org/10.1007/978-3-319-61249-2_3

23

Table 3.1 American Society of Anesthesiology physical status classification [4]

Class	Description	Suitability for sedation
I	A normally healthy patient	Excellent
II	A patient with mild systemic disease	Generally good
III	A patient with severe systemic disease	Intermediate to poor
IV	A patient with severe systemic disease that is a constant threat to life	Poor
V	A moribund patient who is not expected to survive without the operation	Extremely poor
VI	A declared brain-dead patient whose organs are being removed for donor purposes	/

can be performed safely; if the child fits in ASA class III, the benefits of sedation should be carefully weighed against the risk, and anesthesiologist-administered sedation will be preferred. Children in ASA class IV and V must be anesthetized by anesthesiologists.

During the last 10 years many experiences have been reported in adult patients, and reports in children are rising [5]. This situation still remains not ideal and requires future actions to increase the number of anesthesiologists.

3.3   Preparation for Sedation

According to the American Academy of Pediatrics (AAP), health evaluation should be obtained before sedation and include health history, American Society of Anesthesiology score of physical status, medication history, allergy assessment, age, weight, and baseline vital signs (Table 3.2) [6]. Such an evaluation seems to lower the risk of sedation-related complications [7]. A physical exam including the assessment of the heart, circulation, lungs, head, neck, and airway should be performed [6]. Laboratory tests are not required if no specific clinical indications are present. Antibiotic prophylaxis is not necessary for routine endoscopy, even with biopsy [6].

Fast is recommended for a minimum of 2 h from clear liquids, 4 h from breast milk, and 6 h from formula, nonhuman milk and solids before elective sedation [6]. Fast for younger children should be planned with more caution.

Endoscopic procedures should be discussed with parents and children, if emotionally and intellectually competent enough [5]. Premedication with midazolam may be useful for easier intravenous catheter placement and easier separation from parents. Such a premedication procedure is both effective and safe, and both oral and intranasal administration are allowed, even if the last one may cause local discomfort. Intravenous catheter placement is important and should always be secured for administration of sedatives and analgesics (other sedation regimens are less well documented) and intra-procedural emergency events [2, 6].

The AAP recommends continuous pulse oximetry, heart rate and arterial blood pressure monitoring at all levels of sedation [6]. Equipment and supplies for resuscitation should be readily available in any pediatric endoscopy room [5, 8]. The

Table 3.2 Checklist of child's preparation before elective sedation [5]

	Preparation	Comment
Planning of the procedure	Understanding	Explanation of aims and risks
	Informed consent	Signed by parents
	Presedation assessment	Comorbidity
		ASA score (Table 3.1)
		Drugs
		Coagulation
		Previous adverse events to sedation/anesthesia
		Specific contraindications for the planned sedation
Preparation on the day of procedure		Allergies
		The need of antibiotic prophylaxis
		Laboratory tests before the procedure
		Additional important data
	Precise instructions	Fasting time, colon cleansing, etc.
	Focused history	Current health state
		Infectious diseases
		Epidemiologic situation
		Fasting
		Allergy
		Specific contraindications for the planned sedation
	Complete physical examination	Focus on respiratory and cardiovascular systems
	Measurement of baseline vital signs	Arterial blood pressure
		Heart rate
		Pulse oximetry
	Laboratory tests	If needed

ASA American Society of Anesthesiology

personnel have to be trained in pediatric advanced life support maneuvers and have to be ready to face any scenery of complications [1].

3.4   Sedatives for Pediatric Gastrointestinal Endoscopy

The choice of sedatives for pediatric gastrointestinal endoscopy is wide, but affected by two main problems: none of the sedatives commercially available has all the properties of an ideal sedative; the use of many sedatives is "off-label" for children, and medicolegal consequences have to be considered in case of adverse events [5]. The ideal sedative has the following characteristics: predictable dose-dependent level of sedation, rapid onset, broad therapeutic window, anxyolytic effect with anterograde amnesia, absence of undesirable effects, and comfortable recovery without side effects. Literature data propose different molecules, administered either intravenously or orally (Table 3.3). Propofol seems to have the best efficacy and safety profile. Three sedation protocols for pediatric gastrointestinal endoscopy have been recently proposed [5].

Table 3.3 Sedatives for pediatric gastrointestinal endoscopy sedation [5]

Generic name	Mechanism(s) of action	Undesirable effect	Dosage	Time to start/duration
Propofol	GABA receptor agonist; sedation, hypnosis, amnesia	Respiratory depression, apnoea, hypotension, painful injection	<3 years: 2 mg/kg; older children: 1 mg/kg	1–2 min/5–15 min
Ketamine	Binds to the NMDA receptors; anesthesia, analgesia, amnesia, sedation, immobilization	Laryngospasm, hypertension, tachycardia, hypersalivation, vomiting, random movements, emergence phenomena	1–1.5 mg/kg	1–5 min/15 min
Midazolam	GABA receptor agonist; anterograde amnesia, anxiolysis, sedation, hypnosis	Respiratory depression, hypotension, paradoxical agitation	<5 years: 0.05–0.1 mg/kg 6–12 years: 0.025–0.05 mg/kg >12 years: 2–2.5 mg/kg	2–3 min/45–60 min
Fentanyl	Opioid receptors agonist; analgesia and sedation	Respiratory depression, hypotension	1–2 mcg/kg	0.5 min/20–40 min
Sevoflurane	Inhalation anesthetic	Recovery agitation, bradycardia, hypotension, cough, vomiting, seizures	Different concentrations according to the age	
Nitrous oxide	Inhalation anesthetic	Vomiting, dizziness, voice change, euphoria, laughter	Mixture of nitrous oxide (50%) and oxygen	0.5–1 min/5 min

GABA Gamma-aminobutyric acid; *NMDA* N-methyl-D-aspartate

3.4.1 Propofol

Propofol is an anesthetic that exerts its sedative effect by an agonistic action on gamma-aminobutyric acid (GABA) receptors. It is a rapid onset and short-acting anesthetic with a narrow therapeutic range. Propofol has no analgesic properties, so that for painful procedures an analgesic must be added [9]. Propofol is contraindicated in infants younger than 1 month [10]. The usual loading dose of propofol is 2 mg/kg in infants and children younger than 3 years, and 1 mg/kg in older children; subsequent boluses of 1 mg/kg for younger, or 0.5 mg/kg for older children, may be added to ensure the adequate level of sedation. For longer procedures, propofol may be administered in a continuous infusion [9]. To date, propofol is the most promising sedative/anesthetic. The largest multicenter prospective study of propofol sedation for different pediatric procedures evaluated the data of 49,836 propofol sedation episodes and showed that propofol-based sedation is the safest sedation practice for children [8]. Pulmonary aspiration of gastric fluid secondary to vomiting during sedation occurred in four patients, while less serious adverse events occurred with an incidence lower than 150/10000 procedures: desaturation (154), central apnea or upper airway obstruction (124), stridor (10), laryngospasm (20), excessive salivation (73), and vomiting (10). Propofol is rarely used by non-anesthesiologists since the administration of propofol is "off-label" in most cases.

3.4.2 Ketamine

Ketamine is a dissociative anesthetic and analgesic, with an antagonistic action on N-methyl-D-aspartate channel [11]. The usual dose of ketamine is 1–2 mg/kg, administered by slow intravenous injection. The sedative effect lasts 10–15 min. Repeated boluses of 0.5 mg/kg prolong its action. The most frequent undesirable effects are vomiting, hypersalivation, nystagmus, hypertension, tachycardia, skin erythema, and emergence phenomena, such as floating sensations, blurred visions, hallucinations, and delirium. Laryngospasm is uncommon. The anticholinergics could be used to prevent hypersalivation [12], but are no longer routinely recommended [5]. Ondansetron prevents vomiting in some patients [13]; it is administered intravenously at 0.1 mg/kg up to a maximum of 2 mg, with a rapid onset of action in 1–3 min. Ketamine-based sedation is safe and effective in otherwise healthy infants older than 3 months. It is contraindicated in infants younger than 3 months, patients with psychosis, uncontrollable hypertension or hyperthyroidism [5].

3.4.3 Benzodiazepines and Opioids

Midazolam is a short-acting benzodiazepine which is widely used for sedation. It acts as an agonist on GABA receptors, and has anxiolytic, amnesic, sedative, hypnotic, muscle relaxant, and anticonvulsant properties [9]. Midazolam is often administered in combination with opioids, especially meperidine, since monotherapy regimen is not sufficient [5]. Studies on adults have shown that sedation with the combination of midazolam and meperidine is safe [14], but no pediatric data are available. The anxiolytic property of midazolam may be useful as premedication, for instance before the placement of an intravenous line. The major undesirable effects are respiratory depression and hypotension, which are avoidable with appropriate dosing and are reversed by the antagonist flumazenil [9].

Opioids are potent analgesics; the most suitable for sedation is fentanyl, because of rapid onset and short action. Fentanyl must be combined with benzodiazepines, as it has no sedation properties. The combination increases the risk of respiratory depression [9]. Fentanyl is usually administered at 1–2 μg/kg. The analgesic effect lasts 20–40 min. Naloxone reverses opioid side effects and normalizes airway function within 1–2 min of application of 0.1 mg/kg (up to 2 mg) intravenous or intramuscular. Its action lasts for 20–40 min; repeated doses might be needed as most opioids (including fentanyl) action lasts longer [9].

3.4.4   Inhalation Anesthetics

Inhalational anesthetics are represented by sevoflurane and nitrous oxide. Sevoflurane has a good safety profile (low incidence of airway hypersecretion, respiratory depression, or cardiovascular complications) [15], and a shorter recovery time. Nonetheless, its use is limited to anesthesiologists [5, 15]. Nitrous oxide is an inert gas with analgesic, sedative and amnesic properties, and a short duration. In adults, nitrous oxide has been used successfully for proctoscopies and colonoscopies. Michaud et al. [16] reported a good experience with 50% nitrous oxide for gastroscopies and proctosigmoidoscopies in children. They did not evaluate it for ileo-colonoscopy nor compare this type of sedation to other protocols [16]. No newer studies have been carried out on nitrous oxide sedation for gastrointestinal endoscopy in children. It is not routinely recommended in pediatric gastrointestinal endoscopy.

Conclusion

The wide diffusion of diagnostic and therapeutic endoscopic procedures in children has raised the attention on the sedation and analgesia protocols. Propofol offers the best balance between efficacy and safety, but its administration is mostly "off-label" for non-anesthesiologists; ketamine and a combination of a benzodiazepine and an opioid are more frequently used for pediatric patients. General anesthesia by a multidisciplinary team led by an anesthesiologist should be preferred. Because of the shortness of anesthesiologists, the creation of sedation teams led by non-anesthesiologists may represent a valid alternative, to be designed in line with national and institutional regulations. The presence of anesthesiologist remains mandatory in case of deep sedation and rescue procedures.

References

1. ASGE Standards of Practice Committee, Lightdale JR, Acosta R, Shergill AK, et al. Modifications in endoscopic practice for pediatric patients. Gastrointest Endosc. 2014;79:699–710.
2. Ramaiah R, Bhananker S. Pediatric procedural sedation and analgesia outside the operating room: anticipating, avoiding and managing complications. Expert Rev Neurother. 2011;11:755–63.
3. van Beek EJ, Leroy PL. Safe and effective procedural sedation for gastrointestinal endoscopy in children. J Pediatr Gastroenterol Nutr. 2012;54:171–85.
4. Faigel DO, Baron TH, Goldstein JL, et al. Guidelines for the use of deep sedation and anesthesia for GI endoscopy. Gastrointest Endosc. 2002;56:613–7.
5. Orel R, Brecelj J, Dias JA, et al. Review on sedation for gastrointestinal tract endoscopy in children by non-anesthesiologists. World J Gastrointest Endosc. 2015;7:895–911.
6. Cote CJ, Wilson S. Guidelines for monitoring and management of pediatric patients during and after sedation for diagnostic and therapeutic procedures: an update. Pediatrics. 2006;118:2587–602.
7. Hoffman GM, Nowakowski R, Troshynski TJ, et al. Risk reduction in pediatric procedural sedation by application of an American Academy of Pediatrics/American Society of Anesthesiologists process model. Pediatrics. 2002;109:236–43.

8. Cravero JP, Beach ML, Blike GT, et al. Pediatric Sedation Research Consortium. The incidence and nature of adverse events during pediatric sedation/anesthesia with propofol for procedures outside the operating room: a report from the Pediatric Sedation Research Consortium. Anesth Analg. 2009;108:795–804.
9. Sahyoun C, Krauss B. Clinical implications of pharmacokinetics and pharmacodynamics of procedural sedation agents in children. Curr Opin Pediatr. 2012;24:225–32.
10. Shah PS, Shah VS. Propofol for procedural sedation/anaesthesia in neonates. Cochrane Database Syst Rev. 2011;3:CD007248.
11. Brecelj J, Trop TK, Orel R. Ketamine with and without midazolam for gastrointestinal endoscopies in children. J Pediatr Gastroenterol Nutr. 2012;54:748–52.
12. Heinz P, Geelhoed GC, Wee C, Pascoe EM. Is atropine needed with ketamine sedation? A prospective, randomised, double blind study. Emerg Med J. 2006;23:206–9.
13. Langston WT, Wathen JE, Roback MG, Bajaj L. Effect of ondansetron on the incidence of vomiting associated with ketamine sedation in children: a double-blind, randomized, placebo-controlled trial. Ann Emerg Med. 2008;52:30–4.
14. Cohen LB, Wecsler JS, Gaetano JN, et al. Endoscopic sedation in the United States: results from a nationwide survey. Am J Gastroenterol. 2006;101:967–74.
15. Montes RG, Bohn RA. Deep sedation with inhaled sevoflurane for pediatric outpatient gastro-intestinal endoscopy. J Pediatr Gastroenterol Nutr. 2000;31:41–6.
16. Michaud L, Gottrand F, Ganga-Zandzou PS, et al. Nitrous oxide sedation in pediatric patients undergoing gastrointestinal endoscopy. J Pediatr Gastroenterol Nutr. 1999;28:310–4.

Early Onset IBD: Endoscopic Features

4

Serena Arrigo, Sara Signa, and Arrigo Barabino

4.1 Introduction

4.1.1 Definition of Very Early Onset IBD (VEOIBD)

Pediatric onset IBD represents 20–25% of cases of IBD [1]. Age of onset provides information about the type of IBD and its associated genetic features, and led to changes in the classification of pediatric IBD. The Montreal classification [2] originally defined patients with onset of <17 years as a distinct group of pediatric onset IBD patients (A1). The Pediatric Paris modification [3] of the Montreal classification later subdivided pediatric IBD in two age groups: those aged 10–16 years (A1b) and those under 10 years (A1a), named early onset IBD, with unique characteristics. In the last years, an increasing body of evidence is suggesting that children with IBD onset at 0–6 years represent a distinct group of pediatric patients. This age group (some use 0–6 and some 0–5 years as the corresponding cutoff) is named very early onset IBD (VEOIBD), of whom 0–2 years should be termed infantile IBD [4]. An extreme early subgroup, defined neonatal IBD, has been described with severe manifestations during the first 27 days of life [5].

The prevalence of VEOIBD varies among different studies, ranging from 3 to 15% of all pediatric IBD [1, 4, 6]. The prevalence of infantile IBD is lower (1–2%) [1].

Clinical pattern of VEOIBD, in particular infantile IBD, differs from older onset IBD (Table 4.1). Isolated pancolitis, increased severity, aggressive progression, more resistant to many of standard therapy, about 25% has underlying immunodeficiency, stronger family history of IBD are the main characteristics [7]. Genetic susceptibility plays an important role in VEOIBD and addresses the need to recognize monogenic disorders that require different treatment.

S. Arrigo · S. Signa · A. Barabino (✉)
Pediatric Gastroenterology and Endoscopy Unit, G. Gaslini Institute—IRCCS, Genoa, Italy
e-mail: serenaarrigo@gaslini.org; arrigobarabino@gaslini.org

© Springer International Publishing AG, part of Springer Nature 2018
L. Dall'Oglio, C. Romano (eds.), *Endoscopy in Pediatric Inflammatory Bowel Disease*,
https://doi.org/10.1007/978-3-319-61249-2_4

Table 4.1 Features of very early onset and older onset inflammatory bowel disease [6]

	VEOIBD	Older onset (>6 year IBD)
Disease distribution	Predominately colonic Ileal involvement <20% Extensive disease at presentation	Ileocolonic Less extensive disease at presentation
Disease histology	CD: 30–35% UC: 35–39% IC: 11–22%	CD: 55–60% UC: 40–45% IC: 4–10%
Positive familiar history	About 40–50%; consanguinity	About 10–20%
Genetic analysis	Increased prevalence of monogenic disorders in <2 years	Polygenic inheritance
Response to conventional therapy	Decreased	Variable
Needs of surgery	71%	55%

4.2   Endoscopic and Histologic Features

Diagnostic workout and criteria of VEOIBD are the same used for the other pediatric IBD, according to the revised Porto criteria [8] and Paris classification [3].

In particular, Crohn's disease (CD) is defined by the presence of: (1) epithelioid cell granuloma in any one biopsy; (2) in the absence of granuloma, typical endoscopic CD lesions, such as aphthous or deep ulcerations with skip lesions all along the gastrointestinal tract and/or segmental small intestinal findings; (3) perianal disease; and (4) transmural inflammation such as structuring of fistulizing disease. Ulcerative colitis (UC) is defined as continuous disease from the rectum confined to the colon with typical histology. The rectal sparing is diagnostic for UC if it is macroscopic but not microscopic. An inverse correlation between age of onset and frequency of rectal sparing is described [8].

Pediatric IBD often presents as unspecific intestinal inflammation encompassing endoscopic and histological features of both CD and UC [6]. All cases of isolated colitis that could not definitively be declared as CD or UC are defined as IBD-U with features of CD (CD-like) or of UC (UC-like). UC phenotypes could evolve into CD disease. VEOIBD patients are more likely to have their initial diagnosis change throughout their course of illness [9].

All different reports describe a predominant isolated colonic disease at the diagnosis [4, 10]. VEOIBD are more commonly diagnosed with UC (35–59%) as compared to older onset IBD, in which CD is more prevalent (55–60%). The UC extension is similar in the two age groups. Approximately 30–35% of VEOIBD patients are diagnosed with CD, with a colonic involvement, in contrast with older children and adults who have a predominant small bowel or ileocecal disease. IBD-U is diagnosed more often in patients with VEOIBD (11–22%) and declined progressively with increasing age (4–10% in older IBD) [6, 11–15]. It is reported that approximately one fifth of children with IBD under 6 and one third of children with IBD under 3 years of age are labeled as IBD-U, reflecting the aspecificity of clinical, endoscopic and histological findings, as well as a potential bias due to incomplete diagnostic workup in very young children [1].

Infantile IBD is always more commonly restricted to the colon, with high rate of IBD-U (such as 34%, even 71%) [4] and CD-like phenotype [11, 12, 16]. Some authors reported UC also in the first 2 years of life [17].

The presence of eosinophilic infiltrate in the colonic mucosa sometimes represents an isolated and early sign of inflammatory colitis and misleads the diagnosis, since it is present also in other conditions such as allergic colitis due to cow milk allergy, the most common cause of rectal bleeding in the first year of age [1, 18]. Two studies reported a diagnostic delay of at least 6 months in VEOIBD [16].

Neonatal IBD is a very rare intractable ulcerating enterocolitis of infancy [5], first described in 1991 by Sanderson. Inflammation is transmural and pan-enteric, typically with well-circumscribed, deep flat ulceration of the mucosa, often associated to a severe perianal disease and a poor outcome. All described patients had immunological abnormalities, underwent immunosuppressive therapy and colectomy to control symptoms and one third of them developed subsequently a lymphoma. A high incidence of consanguinity is reported.

4.3   Endoscopy and Primary Immunodeficiencies (PID)

Gastrointestinal inflammation due to immune dysregulation can be the initial or leading symptom of PID. In other cases, IBD is the result of an increased susceptibility for infections. The majority of severe PID manifests during early childhood [19]. Over 50 genetic disorders have been identified and associated with IBD-like immunopathology, named monogenic IBD [1].

Defects in every aspect of the immune system, such as neutrophils, T-cell and B-cell lymphocytes, and macrophages, are associated with VEOIBD. Also non-lymphohematopoietic defects with primary defects in enterocytes can also lead IBD-like manifestations. Based on the pathophysiology, VEOIBD can be categorized as [18]:

- Defects in T-cell immune tolerance (IPEX and IPEX-like disorders).
- Defects in IL-10/IL-10 receptor (R) signaling.
- Hyperinflammatory and autoinflammatory disorders (mevalonate kinase deficiency, familial mediterranean fever, XIAP deficiency).
- Defects in neutrophil function (chronic granulomatous disease—CGD; glycogen storage disease type-1b, leucocyte-adhesion deficiency syndromes).
- Defects in epithelial barrier function (NEMO, ADAM17, TTC7A deficiency).
- Isolated or combined T-cell and B-cell defects (common variable immunodeficiency—CVID, hyper-immunoglobulin M syndrome, Hyper IgE syndrome and agammaglobulinemia, Wiskott–Aldrich syndrome—WAS).

IBD in PID are endoscopically and histologically poorly characterized. The few existing case reports show very heterogeneous manifestations of intestinal inflammation which in most cases does not allow a PID diagnosis by itself. The gut endoscopy in polygenic IBD versus monogenic IBD due to PID are indistinguishable. Also, histological findings do generally not allow differentiation between the entities [1].

Table 4.2 When to suspect PID (adapted from [1, 19])

Very early onset	PID with IBD phenotype mainly manifest in very early onset, particularly less than 2 years
Family history	Above all consanguinity, predominance of affected males or multiple family members
Severe disease	Severe disease, severe perianal disease, necessity of parenteral nutrition, steroids, complications, and therapy refractory course
Atypical endoscopic or histopathologic findings	Atypical macroscopic and microscopic findings, e.g., non-celiac villous atrophy or lacking plasma or extreme epithelial apoptosis
Extraintestinal manifestations	Hair/nail/skin dystrophy, granuloma, autoimmunity, tumors
Recurrent or unusual infections	Many PID show an increased susceptibility for severe, prolonged, opportunistic or recurrent infections and fever or macrophage activation syndrome
Abnormal blood tests	Neutro-/lymphopenia, reduced mean platelet volume (MPV), abnormal immunoglobulin levels or lymphocyte subsets

Endoscopy can show a severe ulcerative inflammation in the colon mimicking CD in some cases of NEMO and LBRA deficiency, in about 40% of patients with CGD, and in about 20% of XIAP deficiency. NCF2 deficiency is a variant of CGD and can appear with an infantile colitis, severe fistulizing perianal and structuring disease. IBD-like features above all CD-like are described in glycogen storage disease type 1b. A IL-10/IL-10R deficiency causes an infantile severe discontinuous ulcerative IBD (colitis or ileocolitis) with pronounced perianal disease and fistulas. Histology shows granulomas (often multiple, well-formed and with no inflammatory change), pigmented macrophages and nonspecific chronic inflammation above all the colon in CGD, crypt abscesses indistinct from IBD and sometimes apoptosis in XIAP, abscesses and granulomas or nonspecific neutrophilic infiltrate in IL-10/IL-10R defects [6, 19]. Villous atrophy may be present in NEMO deficiency [6]. In TTC7A, varying degrees of intestinal atresia are reported.

In WAS are described CD-like process with cobblestone appearance and inflammatory pseudopolyps as well UC-like features [6].

CVID can cause aphthous lesions in the colon and histological autoimmune colitis with multiple apoptosis and cryptitis and typical low or absence of plasma cells. Enteropathy with villous atrophy, mimicking celiac disease, with low or absent plasma cells can be associated [19].

Villous atrophy with lymphocytic and eosinophilic infiltration, apoptosis of epithelial cells and antienterocyte antibodies is present in IPEX (-like) enteropathy, mimicking a graft-versus-host disease and autoimmune enteropathy [6, 19]. Colitis with bloody diarrhea can be associated [6].

In summary, endoscopic and histological features of PID-associated IBD are insufficient to either confirm or exclude an underlying PID, but play a central role in characterizing the suspected PID and determine the extension and severity of the IBD [19].

Anamnestic and clinical data and immunologic laboratory tests are of paramount importance for the diagnostic workup (Table 4.2). Despite not routinary, genetic screening using next-generation sequencing (NGS) and/or whole-exome sequencing (WES) represents an important tool to identify the monogenic defect [1, 20, 21].

4.4   Clinical Presentation and Course of VEOIBD

Rectal bleeding and bloody diarrhea are the most common symptoms at VEOIBD diagnosis, reflecting a colonic location [4]. Abdominal pain seems to be less common than older IBD. Significant weight loss and systemic symptoms like recurrent fever are prevalent in younger and in CD and IBD-U phenotype. Perianal disease could be present at the diagnosis, with perineal erythema, fissures, and voluminous tags until fistula and abscess. An acronym used to remember all the clinical key features that may lead to a diagnosis of PID is YOUNG AGE MATTERS MOST [1]: YOUNG AGE onset, Multiple family members and consanguinity, Autoimmunity, Thriving failure, Treatment with conventional medication fails, Endocrine concerns, Recurrent infections or unexplained fever, Severe perianal disease, Macrophage activation syndrome and hemophagocytic lymphohistiocytosis, Obstruction and atresia of intestine, Skin lesions and dental and hair abnormalities, and Tumors [1, 19, 22].

Extraintestinal manifestation rates at diagnosis are similar between VEOIBD, EOIBD, and older groups [23, 24].

Pediatric Ulcerative Colitis Activity Index (PUCAI) and Pediatric Crohn Disease Activity Index (PCDAI) are useful tools also in very young children [23]. ANCA and ASCA are not helpful in the diagnosis of VEOIBD, in contrast to older children with IBD [12].

In children younger of 1 year of age, colitis can have an insidious course variable from mild symptoms to severe colitis [18]. In this age, cow's milk protein allergy is common and a trial of elimination diet is a customary treatment [1, 17]. However, food intolerance and allergy can be secondary to the disorder and allergen avoidance could also alleviate the inflammation of classic IBD [1]. A diagnosis of infantile IBD should be considered in the absence of response to dietary modification and profound impact of the disease on weight and growth, as well as in the presence of other IBD-associated features such as perianal involvement [16].

Treatment for VEOIBD is the same as that given to adolescents and adults with IBD (e.g., anti-inflammatory agents, immunomodulators, biologics, antibiotics, and surgical approaches) [7]. The clinical course of VEOIBD patients can be either refractory or responsive also to first-line treatment, such as mesalamine [4, 25].

The majority of patients with the IBD onset in the first 1–2 years of age can have a serious evolution requiring parenteral nutrition, early use of immunosuppressors and until one third of them requires surgical treatment, as colectomy or ileal diversion to control the disease [26]. It is important to have a high index of suspicion for monogenic forms in VEOIBD because the likelihood is estimated as high as 25–30%, especially in the infantile IBD, in severe cases and in significant perianal disease [4]. Identification of a specific monogenic defect might lead to more of a precision medicine approach, including stem-cell transplantation (HSCT), antibiotics, abatacept therapy, or other therapies [7].

Conclusions

VEOIBD refers to a subgroup of pediatric IBD diagnosed before 6 years of age. This subgroup differs from adolescent and adult disease as it is usually restricted to the colon and refractory to medical treatments. Nonetheless, not all VEOIBD has a poor prognosis.

Up to 25% of VEOIBD has an identified underlying immunodeficiency, especially in case of: age onset less 2 years (infantile IBD), aggressive course and progression, resistance to medical treatment, strong family history of IBD, and other specific features as infections. Specific mutations in IL-10/IL-10R, NCF2, XIAP, FOXP3, LRBA, ADAM17, and TTC7A have been identified.

The detection of PID opens the way to more targeted therapy, such as HSCT, and assesses the prognosis. To date, genetic screening (NGS, WES, and even whole genome sequencing) can help in the identification of an underlying genetic defect.

Unless the patient clearly has one of the rare mutations mentioned above, treatment for VEOIBD is the same of older onset disease.

References

1. Uhlig HH, Schwerd T, Koletzko S, Shah N, Kammermeier J, Elkadri A, et al. The diagnostic approach to monogenic very early onset inflammatory bowel disease. Gastroenterology. 2014;147:990–1007.
2. Silverberg MS, Satsangi J, Ahmad T, Arnott ID, Bernstein CN, Brant S, et al. Toward an integrated clinical, molecular and serological classification of inflammatory bowel disease: report of a Working Party of the 2005 Montreal World Congress of Gastroenterology. Can J Gastroenterol. 2005;19(Suppl A):5A–36A.
3. Levine A, Griffiths A, Markowitz J, Wilson DC, Turner D, Russell RK, et al. Pediatric modification of the Montreal classification for inflammatory bowel disease: the Paris classification. Inflamm Bowel Dis. 2011;17:1314–21.
4. Turner D, Muise AM. Very early onset IBD: how very different 'on average'? J Crohns Colitis. 2017;11:517–8.
5. Thapar N, Shah N, Ramsay AD, Lindley KJ, Milla PJ. Long-term outcome of intractable ulcerating enterocolitis of infancy. J Pediatr Gastroenterol Nutr. 2005;40:582–8.
6. Kelsen JR, Baldassano RN, Artis D, Sonnenberg GF. Maintaining intestinal health: the genetics and immunology of very early onset inflammatory bowel disease. Cell Mol Gastroenterol Hepatol. 2015;1(1):462–76.
7. Snapper SB. Very-early-onset inflammatory bowel disease. Gastroenterol Hepatol (N Y). 2015;11:554–6.
8. Levine A, Koletzko S, Turner D, Escher JC, Cucchiara S, de Ridder L, et al. ESPGHAN revised Porto group for the diagnosis of inflammatory bowel disease in children and adolescents. J Pediatr Gastroenterol Nutr. 2014;58:795–806.
9. Benchimol EI, Mack DR, Nguyen GC, et al. Incidence, outcomes, and health services burden of very early onset inflammatory bowel disease. Gastroenterology. 2014;147:803–13.
10. Capriati T, Cardile S, Papadatou B, Romano C, Knafelz D, Bracci F, et al. Pediatric inflammatory bowel disease. Specificity of very early onset. Expert Rev Clin Immunol. 2016;12:963–72.

11. Heyman MB, Kirschner BS, Gold BD, Ferry G, Baldassano R, Cohen SA, et al. Children with early-onset inflammatory bowel disease (IBD): analysis of a pediatric IBD consortium registry. J Pediatr. 2005;146:35–40.
12. Mamula P, Telega GW, Markowitz JE, et al. Inflammatory bowel disease in children 5 years of age and younger. Am J Gastroenterol. 2002;97:2005–10.
13. Aloi M, Lionetti P, Barabino A, et al. Phenotype and disease course of early-onset pediatric inflammatory bowel disease. Inflamm Bowel Dis. 2014;20:597–605.
14. Oliva-Hemker M, Hutfless S, Al Kazzi ES, Lerer T, Mack D, LeLeiko N, et al. Clinical presentation and five-year therapeutic management of very early-onset inflammatory bowel disease in a large North American cohort. J Pediatr. 2015;167:527–32.
15. Bequet E, Sarter H, Fumery M, Vasseur F, Armengol-Debeir L, Pariente B, et al. Incidence and phenotype at diagnosis of very-early-onset compared with later-onset paediatric inflammatory bowel disease: a population-based study [1988-2011]. J Crohns Colitis. 2017;11:519–26.
16. Kammermeier J, Dziubak R, Pescarin M, Drury S, Godwin H, Reeve K, et al. Phenotypic and genotypic characterization of inflammatory bowel disease presenting before the age of 2 years. J Crohn Colitis. 2017;11:60–9.
17. Cannioto Z, Berti I, Martelossi S, Bruno I, Giurici N, Crovella S, et al. IBD and IBD mimicking enterocolitis in children younger than 2 years of age. Eur J Pediatr. 2009;168:149–55.
18. Chandrakasan S, Venkateswaran S, Kugathasan S. Nonclassic inflammatory bowel disease in young infants: immune dysregulation, polyendocrinopathy, enteropathy, X-linked syndrome, and other disorders. Pediatr Clin N Am. 2017;64:139–60.
19. Tegtmeyer D, Seidl M, Gerner P, Baumann U, Klemann C. IBD due to PID: inflammatory bowel disease caused by primary immunodeficiencies—clinical presentations, review of literature, and proposal of a rational diagnostic algorithm. Pediatr Allergy Immunol. 2017;28(5):412–29. https://doi.org/10.1111/pai.12734.
20. Bianco AM, Girardelli M, Tommasini A. Genetics of inflammatory bowel disease from multifactorial to monogenic forms. World J Gastroenterol. 2015;21:12296–310.
21. Moran CJ, Klein C, Muise AM, Snapper SB. Very early-onset inflammatory bowel disease: gaining insight through focused discovery. Inflamm Bowel Dis. 2015;21:1166–75.
22. Girardelli M, Arrigo S, Barabino A, Loganes C, Morreale G, Crovella S, et al. The diagnostic challenge of very-early-onset enterocolitis in an infant with XIAP deficiency. BMC Pediatr. 2015;15:208.
23. Ledder O, Catto-Smith AG, Oliver MR, Alex G, Cameron DJ, Hardikar W. Clinical patterns and outcome of early-onset inflammatory bowel disease. J Pediatr Gastroenterol Nutr. 2014;59:562–4.
24. Gupta N, Bostrom AG, Kirschner BS, Cohen SA, Abramson O, Ferry GD, et al. Presentation and disease course in early- compared to later-onset pediatric Crohn's disease. Am J Gastroenterol. 2008;108:2092–8.
25. Marx G, Seidman EG, Martin SR, Deslandres C. Outcome of Crohn's disease diagnosed before two years of age. J Pediatr. 2002;140:470–3.
26. Ruemmele FM, El Khoury MG, Talbotec C, Maurage C, Mougenot JF, Schmitz J, et al. Characteristics of inflammatory bowel disease with onset during the first year of life. J Pediatr Gastroenterol Nutr. 2006;43:603–9.

Esophagogastroduodenoscopy and Ileocolonoscopy

5

Massimo Martinelli, Caterina Strisciuglio, and Erasmo Miele

5.1 Introduction

Ileocolonoscopy and esophagogastroduodenoscopy (EGD) are recommended as the initial workup for all children with suspected IBD [1]. Endoscopy remains the corner stone in the diagnosis and management of IBD, with several endpoints: (a) differential diagnosis between IBD and other conditions, and between Crohn's disease (CD) and ulcerative colitis (UC) (2); (b) assessing disease location and extent, and efficacy of medical therapy; (c) risk for postsurgical recurrence monitoring; (d) therapeutic role, in case of strictures and bleeding; and (e) cancer surveillance.

5.2 Upper Gastrointestinal Endoscopy

EGD should be performed as part of the first-line investigation in all cases of suspected IBD [1, 2]. Multiple biopsies (2 or more) per section from the esophagus, stomach, and duodenum should be obtained, even in the absence of macroscopic lesions. Absence of specific upper gastrointestinal symptoms, such as dysphagia, pain when eating, nausea and/or vomiting, and aphthous lesions of the mouth, does not preclude the presence of upper gastrointestinal inflammation [3].

M. Martinelli, M.D. · E. Miele, M.D., Ph.D. (✉)
Department of Translational Medical Science, Section of Pediatrics, University of Naples "Federico II", Naples, Italy
e-mail: erasmo.miele@unina.it

C. Strisciuglio, M.D., Ph.D.
Department of Woman, Child and General and Specialized Surgery, Second University of Naples, Caserta, Italy

© Springer International Publishing AG, part of Springer Nature 2018
L. Dall'Oglio, C. Romano (eds.), *Endoscopy in Pediatric Inflammatory Bowel Disease*, https://doi.org/10.1007/978-3-319-61249-2_5

5.2.1 Crohn's Disease

UGI involvement seems to be more common in children with CD, when compared to adult CD patients. The Paris classification, validated in 2011 from Montreal classification, introduced the separation within L4 class in patients with an upper gastrointestinal (UGI) involvement proximal (L4a) or distal to Treitz ligament (L4b) [4] (Table 5.1). Macroscopic UGI lesions are reported in 2.4–8.8% CD adult patients [5–7]. Data from the German-language CEDATA-GPGE registry, including 616 children with CD, showed lesions in the UGI tract in approximately half of patients, and 7.2% of them had also an involvement of the small intestine [8]. Similarly, the EUROKIDS Registry, an inception cohort including 1811 untreated pediatric IBD patients evaluated at diagnosis, reported a macroscopic involvement of the UGI tract in 35% of CD children, of whom 24% were specific for CD (aphthae, ulcerations, cobblestoning, and stenosis) [9]. Endoscopic findings in UGI in patients with CD are reported in Table 5.2.

Microscopic mucosal lesions have been reported in biopsies from the UGI in 64–90% of patients with CD and in 38–70% of patients with UC [10]. The isolated detection of epithelioid granulomas, the histological hallmark of gastric CD, in pediatric patients with CD, ranges from 2 to 21% [11]. Other histological findings are nonspecific and not helpful in discriminating CD from UC. Focally enhanced gastritis (FEG), characterized by a focal pit or gland inflammation consisting of lymphocytes and macrophage resulting in epithelial injury, and focal cryptitis of the duodenum are significantly more present in patients with CD compared with children with non-IBD, but not with children with UC [10, 12]. Among CD patients, FEG seems to be more common in younger patients with peak in the 5–10-year-old age group [13].

Table 5.1 Paris classification for pediatric Crohn's disease

Age at diagnosis
  A1a: 0–<10 year
  A1b: 10–<17 year
  A2: 17–40 year
Location
  L1: distal 1/3 ileal ± limited cecal disease
  L2: colonic
  L3: ileocolonic
  L4a: upper disease proximal to ligament of Treitz
  L4b: upper disease distal to ligament of Treitz and proximal to distal 1/3 ileum
Behavior
  B1: non-stricturing non-penetrating
  B2: stricturing
  B3: penetrating
  B2 B3: both penetrating and stricturing disease, either at the same or different times
  p: perianal disease modifier
Growth
  G0: no evidence of growth delay
  G1: growth delay

Table 5.2 Endoscopic findings of the upper GI tract in Crohn's disease	Esophagus	Erythema
		Erosions
		Ulcers
		Polypoid lesions
		Pseudomembranous formations
		Strictures
		Mucosal bridges
		Perforations
		Fistulas
	Stomach and duodenum	Superficial ulcers
		Aphthous ulcers
		Linear ulcers
		Serpiginous ulcers
		Nodularity
		Cobblestone appearance
		Rigidity of the GI wall
		Narrowing of the lumen

5.2.2 Ulcerative Colitis

The revised Porto criteria have recently added UGI involvement within UC phenotypes [1]. Several studies have demonstrated that macroscopic and histological lesions in UGI are present both in pediatric and adult patients with UC [11, 14–17] (Fig. 5.1a, b). Mild ulceration and microscopic involvement of the UGI are reported in 4–8% of pediatric and adult UC patients [18]. The EUROKIDS Registry showed that UGI involvement occurred in 4% of UC children. Erosions in the stomach were present in 3.1% of UC children, while frank ulcerations in 0.4%; erosions or ulcerations limited to the esophagus or duodenum were detected in 0.8% [8].

5.3 Lower Endoscopy

Ileocolonoscopy represents the most powerful diagnostic tool for suspected IBD. On the basis of the revised Porto criteria and the ECCO-based consensus for endoscopy in IBD, ileocolonoscopy with biopsies is the preferred procedure to establish the diagnosis and extent of disease [1, 19]. It is recommended to perform it soon after patient referral and possibly before the initiation of any medical treatment [1, 19].

5.3.1 Crohn's Disease

5.3.1.1 Diagnosis

The classical macroscopic pattern of pediatric CD is characterized by the patchy distribution of inflammation with skip lesions (areas of inflammation interposed between normal appearing mucosa), aphthous ulcers, and cobblestoning (Fig. 5.2) [19]. Aphthous ulcerations are usually the earliest lesions [20], and together with the evidence of linear or serpiginous ulcers the diagnosis of CD

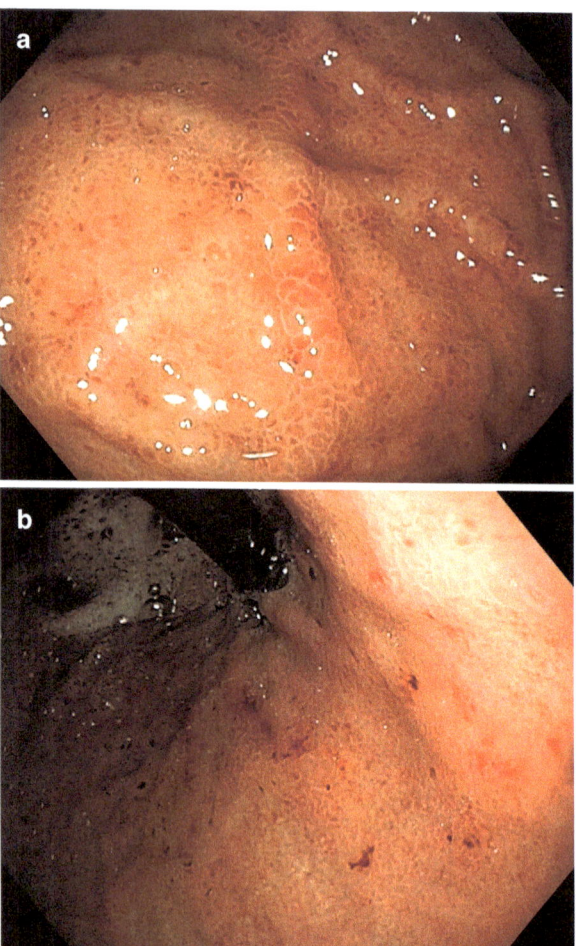

should be strongly suspected. Cobblestoning derives from interception of long ulcerative and large tortuous lesions with areas of thickened mucosa within it [1]. About the vascular pattern, CD children usually show a patchy involvement of vascular architecture, with normal areas surrounded by areas characterized by the total absence of vessels [19]. The evidence of strictures or fistulas during the performance of ileocolonoscopy should be considered as an almost pathognomonic CD sign [1].

5.3.1.2 Disease Location and Extent

The current accepted classification for location and extent of disease is the Paris classification (Table 5.1) [4]. Pediatric Crohn's disease is divided in: ileal (L1), colonic (L2), ileocolonic (L3), and UGI involvement (L4a and L4b). As in adults, pediatric CD may involve any area of the GI tract but, differently from adults, the

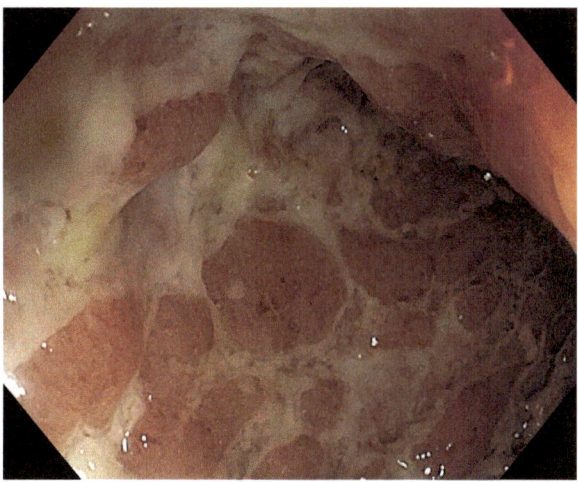

Fig. 5.2 Endoscopic features of Crohn's disease

main CD presentation in pediatric age remains still the ileocolonic involvement (53%) [21]. In younger patients, particularly those <2 years of age in whom colonic disease is prominent, differential diagnosis with UC is usually more difficult, with a higher number of IBD-unclassified diagnosis [1].

5.3.2   Ulcerative Colitis

5.3.2.1 Diagnosis

UC endoscopic classical pattern is characterized also in pediatric age by erythema and vascular congestion. The mucosa is typically very friable and easily bleeding at minor contact on various degrees, depending on the activity of disease and leading to the formation of ulcers (Fig. 5.3) [1, 20]. A classical "granular" appearance may be identified when edema is prominent. Mucosal atrophy may be identified as a consequence of chronic inflammation and is thought to be a possible trigger of pseudopolyps. Pseudopolyps represent another UC landmark, caused by the attempt of regeneration of previously ulcerated areas. It usually appears as long, fingerlike projections, with different shapes. It is usually recommended to obtain biopsies from them, although they are not classically associated with malignancies [19]. As described in the revised Porto criteria [1], atypical endoscopic patterns exist. The main atypical UC morphology may be found in children presenting with the "so-called" Acute Severe colitis (ASC) [1]. The severity of inflammation leads to a transmural involvement and to the formation of deep ulcers [1], easily misdiagnosed with Crohn's colitis.

5.3.2.2 Disease Location and Extent

UC has typically been described as a chronic continuous mucosal inflammation within the colonic segments. On the basis of the recent Paris classification, pediatric UC inflammation may be confined to the rectum (proctitis), from the rectum up to the splenic flexure (left-side colitis), beyond the splenic flexure (extensive

Fig. 5.3 Endoscopic features of severe ulcerative colitis

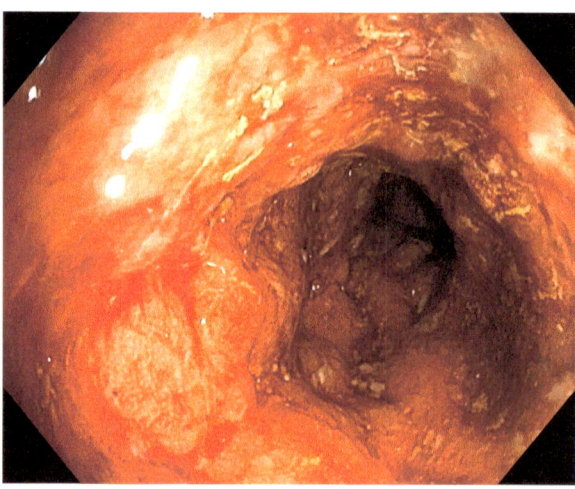

Table 5.3 Paris classification for pediatric ulcerative colitis

Extent of disease
　E1: ulcerative proctitis
　E2: left-side colitis (distal to splenic flexure)
　E3: extensive colitis (distal to hepatic flexure)
　E4: pancolitis (proximal to hepatic flexure)
Severity of disease
　S0: never severe
　S1[a]: severe

[a]Severe defined by Pediatric Ulcerative Colitis Activity Index (PUCAI)

colitis), or may include the entire colon (pancolitis) [4] (Table 5.3). The recently revised Porto criteria have shed light on atypical pediatric UC locations [1], among which rectal sparing and cecal patch are the best known [1]. Rectal sparing is characterized by a various colonic involvement, with the sparing of rectal tract. In children, it has been reported in 5–30% at diagnosis, and it is usually more frequent among younger children [9, 22]. In adult UC, it has generally been associated to the use of topical therapy [23]. Cecal patch has been described in 2% of UC children at diagnosis [9] and is characterized by the concomitant presence of a mild degree of inflammation in left-sided colon and in cecum, classically around the periappendiceal region.

5.4   Follow-Up

Once an IBD diagnosis has been established, ileocolonoscopy keeps its fundamental role during the follow-up of the patients in evaluating the relapse of disease, the need for new treatment strategies, the cancer surveillance and, based on the most recent evidences, the response to therapy [19]. Referring to the most recent ECCO guidelines, endoscopic reassessment should always be considered in cases of:

– Relapse and flare of disease, in order to differentiate IBD relapse versus a super-imposed infection, such as clostridium difficile [1].
– Modifications of therapy.
– Refractoriness.
– New symptoms.
– Patients undergoing surgery: ileocolonoscopy is the gold standard in the diagnosis of CD postoperative recurrence. It is recommended 6–12 months after surgery where treatment decisions may be affected [19]. Indeed, the endoscopic appearance 6–12 months after the surgery is useful to estimate relapse risk and orientate postoperative treatment [19, 24]. Endoscopy is also indicated in the IBD patients undergoing ileal pouch anal anastomosis (IPAA) for the monitoring of pouchitis development. In case of suggestive symptoms, colonoscopy with biopsies should be performed [19].
– Longstanding UC and CD colitis, to monitor the development of dysplasia and colorectal cancer (CRC) [19].

It is still debated the real need to evaluate the response to therapy in a patient with quiescent disease. Increasing evidence suggests that mucosal healing should be considered as the essential outcome of medical treatment of both UC and CD [25–27]. Conversely, the most recent ECCO guidelines on endoscopy in IBD still stated that routine endoscopy for patients in clinical remission is unnecessary, unless it is likely to change management [19]. The reason is that prognostic implications of endoscopic reevaluation in quiescent disease have not yet been determined and investigated [19].

References

1. Levine A, Koletzko S, Turner D, et al. ESPGHAN revised porto criteria for the diagnosis of inflammatory bowel disease in children and adolescents. J Pediatr Gastroenterol Nutr. 2014;58:795–806.
2. Bousvarous A, Antonioli DA, Colletti RB, et al. Differentiating ulcerative colitis from Crohn disease in children and young adults: report of a working group of the North American Society for Pediatric Gastroenterology, Hepatology, and Nutrition and the Crohn's and Colitis Foundation of America. J Pediatr Gastroenterol Nutr. 2007;44:653–74.
3. D'Haens G, Rutgeerts P, Geboes K, Vantrappen G. The natural history of esophageal Crohn's disease: three patterns of evolution. Gastrointest Endosc. 1994;40:296–300.
4. Levine A, Griffiths A, Markowitz J, et al. Pediatric modification of the Montreal classification for inflammatory bowel disease: the Paris classification. Inflamm Bowel Dis. 2011;17:1314–21.
5. Nguyen GC, Torres EA, Requeiro M. Inflammatory bowel disease characteristics among Africans, Americans, Hispanics, and non-Hispanic Whites: characterization of a large North American cohort. Am J Gastroenterol. 2006;101:1012–23.
6. Vind I, Riis L, Jess T, et al. Increasing in incidences of inflammatory bowel disease and decreasing surgery rates in Copenhagen City and county, 2003–2005: a population-based study from the Danish Crohn colitis database. Am J Gastroenterol. 2006;101:1274–82.
7. Jess T, Riis L, Vind I, et al. Changes in clinical characteristics, course, and prognosis of inflammatory bowel disease during the last 5 decades: a population-based study from Copenhagen, Denmark. Inflamm Bowel Dis. 2007;13:481–9.
8. Buderus S, Scholz D, Behrens R, et al. Inflammatory bowel disease in pediatric patients—characteristics of newly diagnosed patients from the CEDATA-GPGE registry. Dtsch Arztebl Int. 2015;112:121–7.

9. Levine A, de Bie CL, Turner D, et al. Atypical disease phenotypes in paediatric ulcerative colitis: 5-year analyses of the EUROKIDS registry. Inflamm Bowel Dis. 2013;19:370–7.

10. Hummel TZ, ten Kate FJ, Reitsma JB, Benninga MA, Kindermann A. Additional value of upper GI tract endoscopy in the diagnostic assessment of childhood IBD. J Pediatr Gastroenterol Nutr. 2012;54(6):753–7.

11. Paerregaard A. What does the IBD patient hide in the upper gastrointestinal tract? Inflamm Bowel Dis. 2009;15:1101–4.

12. Goldstein N, Dulai M. Contemporary morphologic definition of backwash ileitis in ulcerative colitis and features that distinguish it from Crohn disease. Am J Clin Pathol. 2006;126:365–76.

13. Ushiku T, Moran CJ, Lauwers GY. Focally enhanced gastritis in newly diagnosed pediatric inflammatory bowel disease. Am J Surg Pathol. 2013;37:1882–8.

14. Tobin JM, Sinha B, Ramani P, et al. Upper gastrointestinal mucosal disease in pediatric Crohn disease and ulcerative colitis: a blinded, controlled study. J Pediatr Gastroenterol Nutr. 2001;32:443–8.

15. Castellaneta SP, Afzalna GM, et al. Diagnostic role of upper endoscopy in pediatric inflammatory bowel disease. J Pediatr Gastroenterol Nutr. 2004;39:257–61.

16. Abdullah BA, Gupta SK, Croffie JN, et al. The role of esophagogastroduodenoscopy in the initial evaluation of childhood inflammatory bowel disease a 7-year study. J Pediatr Gastroenterol Nutr. 2002;35:636–40. 7.

17. Sawczenko A, Sandhu BK. Presenting features of inflammatory bowel disease in Great Britain and Ireland. Arch Dis Child. 2003;88:995–1000.

18. Robert ME, Tang L, Hao LM, et al. Patterns of inflammation in mucosal biopsies of ulcerative colitis: perceived differences in pediatric populations are limited to children younger than 10 years. Am J Surg Pathol. 2004;28:183–9.

19. Annese V, Daperno M, Rutter MD, et al. European evidence based consensus for endoscopy in inflammatory bowel disease. J Crohns Colitis. 2013;7:982–1018.

20. Chan G, Fefferman DS, Farrell RJ. Endoscopic assessment of inflammatory bowel disease: colonoscopy/esophagogastroduodenoscopy. Gastroenterol Clin N Am. 2012;41:271–90.

21. deBie CI, Paerregaard A, Kolacek S, et al. Disease phenotype at diagnosis in pediatric Crohn's disease: 5-year analyses of the EUROKIDS Registry. Inflamm Bowel Dis. 2013;19:378–85.

22. Rajwal SR, Puntis JW, McClean P, et al. Endoscopic rectal sparing in children with untreated ulcerative colitis. J Pediatr Gastroenterol Nutr. 2004;38:66–9.

23. Odze R, Antonioli D, Peppercorn M, Goldman H. Effect of topical 5-aminosalicylic acid (5-ASA) therapy on rectal mucosal biopsy morphology in chronic ulcerative colitis. Am J Surg Pathol. 1993;17:869–75.

24. Hanauer SB, Korelitz BI, Rutgeerts P, Peppercorn MA, Thisted RA, Cohen RD, et al. Postoperative maintenance of Crohn's disease remission with 6-mercaptopurine, mesalamine, or placebo: a 2-year trial. Gastroenterology. 2004;127:723–9.

25. Rutgeerts P, Vermeire S, Van Assche G. Mucosal healing in inflammatory bowel disease: impossible ideal or therapeutic target? Gut. 2007;56:453–5.

26. Colombel JF, Rutgeerts P, Reinisch W, Esser D, Wang Y, Lang Y, et al. Early mucosal healing with infliximab is associated with improved long-term clinical outcomes in ulcerative colitis. Gastroenterology. 2011;141:1194–201.

27. Peyrin-Biroulet L, Sandborn W, Sands BE, et al. Selecting therapeutic targets in inflammatory bowel disease (STRIDE): determining therapeutic goals for treat-to-target. Am J Gastroenterol. 2015;110:1324–38.

Endoscopic Score in CD and UC

6

Salvatore Oliva

6.1 Introduction

The scoring of endoscopic disease activity is becoming an important clinical end-point in clinical trials [1–3]. The distribution and severity of inflammation noted during endoscopy of children early in the course of IBD may be patchy, with a pattern that is less commonly seen in adults with IBD. For this reason, scoring systems used in adults may not be easily extrapolated to children. Reporting of endoscopic disease activity should always include accurate descriptors of any abnormalities in each segment [4]. It is recommended to use scores in clinical practice but, generally, documentation of endoscopic disease activity remains subjective in children. If endoscopic scoring systems are not used, it is important to report in each segment of the bowel: the extent and location of inflammation; if bowel involvement is continuous or involves skip areas; the presence of erythema, loss of vascular pattern; bleeding (contact or spontaneous); presence of erosions or ulceration (superficial or deep); and the presence of strictures or fistulas. In addition, on follow-up endoscopy, it is important to note the degree of change of endoscopic activity since previous valuation.

A wider application of the scoring system and the development of newer scores will help with the comparison between drug efficacies and optimize a treat-to-target treatment algorithm in management of pediatric IBD patients.

S. Oliva
Pediatric Gastroenterology and Liver Unit, Department of Pediatrics,
Sapienza – University of Rome, Rome, Italy
e-mail: salvatore.oliva@uniroma1.it

© Springer International Publishing AG, part of Springer Nature 2018
L. Dall'Oglio, C. Romano (eds.), *Endoscopy in Pediatric Inflammatory Bowel Disease*,
https://doi.org/10.1007/978-3-319-61249-2_6

6.2   Ulcerative Colitis

Currently there are no validated scoring systems of endoscopic activity for pediatric patients with UC. Definitions of endoscopic disease activity (remission, mild, moderate, and severe disease) and the ability of specific indices to reliably detect meaningful endoscopic changes have either not been rigorously validated or are not available. Some indices form part of composite scores that integrate clinical information (e.g., the Mayo endoscopic sub-score, the Ulcerative Colitis Disease Activity Index). In addition, clinical, endoscopic, and histologic assessments of activity do not always correlate. Furthermore, most scoring systems use the appearance of the rectosigmoid mucosa rather than the entire colon, and do not take segmental differences throughout the colon into consideration, including endoscopic rectal sparing.

Despite the relative simplicity of scoring and category definitions, intra-observer and inter-observer differences among experts remain a significant weakness of current scoring systems. A comprehensive summary of all scoring sheets for CD and UC is shown in Table 6.1.

Table 6.1 Characteristics of the most commonly used scores for UC and CD

Score	Applicability	Variable	Grading
Mayo endoscopic sub-score	UC	Mayo 0	Normal or healed mucosa
		Mayo 1	Faded vascular pattern, mild friability, erythema
		Mayo 2	Absence of vascular pattern, marked friability, erosions
		Mayo 3	Spontaneous bleeding, large ulcers
UCEIS	UC	Vascular pattern	Normal (1): Normal vascular pattern with arborization of capillaries clearly defined
			Patchy loss (2): Patchy loss or blurring of vascular pattern
			Obliterated (3): Complete loss of vascular pattern
		Bleeding	None (1): No visible blood
			Mucosal (2): Some spots or streaks of coagulated blood on the surface of the mucosa ahead of the scope, which can be washed away
			Luminal mild (3): Some free liquid blood in the lumen
			Luminal severe (4): Frank blood in the lumen ahead of endoscope or visible oozing from mucosa after washing intraluminal blood, or visible oozing from a hemorrhagic mucosa
		Erosions and ulcers	None (1): Normal mucosa, no visible erosions or ulcers
			Erosions (2): Tiny ($\leq$5 mm) defects in the mucosa, of a white or yellow color with a flat edge
			Superficial ulcer (3): Larger (>5 mm) defects in the mucosa, which are discrete fibrin-covered ulcers in comparison with erosions, but remain superficial
			Deep ulcer (4): Deeper excavated defects in the mucosa, with a slightly raised edge

Table 6.1 (continued)

Score	Applicability	Variable	Grading
UCCIS	UC	Vascular pattern	0: Normal, clear vascular pattern 1: Partially visible vascular pattern 2: Complete loss of vascular pattern
		Granularity	0: Normal, smooth, and glistening 1: Fine 2: Coarse
		Ulceration	0: Normal, no erosion or ulcer 1: Erosions or pinpoint ulcerations 2: Numerous shallow ulcers with mucopus 3: Deep, excavated ulcerations 4: Diffusely ulcerated with >30% involvement
		Bleeding/friability	0: Normal, no bleeding, no friability 1: Friable, bleeding to light touch 2: Spontaneous bleeding
		Grading of SAES and GAES	0: Normal/quiescent: visible vascular pattern with no bleeding, erosions, ulcers or friability (includes altered vascular pattern in quiescent disease) 1: Mild: erythema, decreased or loss of vascular pattern, fine granularity, but no friability or spontaneous bleeding 2: Moderate: friability with bleeding to light touch, coarse granularity, erosions, or pinpoint ulcerations 3: Severe: spontaneous bleeding or gross ulcers The GAES also includes a 10 cm visual analogue scale of severity. Abbreviations: GAES, global assessment of endoscopic severity; SAES, segmental assessment of endoscopic activity
Rutgeerts score	Postoperative CD	i0	No lesions in the distal ileum
		i1	Less than 5 aphthous lesions in the distal ileum
		i2	>5 aphthous lesions with normal mucosa between the lesions, or skip area of large lesions or lesions confined to ileocolonic anastomosis
		i3	Diffuse aphthous ileitis with extensively inflamed mucosa
		i4	Diffuse inflammation with large ulcers, nodules, and/or stenosis
Modified Rutgeerts score	Postoperative CD	i0	No lesions in the distal ileum
		i1	Less than 5 aphthous lesions in the distal ileum
		i2	>5 aphthous lesions with normal mucosa between the lesions, or skip area of large lesions or lesions confined to ileocolonic anastomosis
		i2a	Lesions confined to the ileocolonic anastomosis (including anastomosis stenosis)
		i2b	More than 5 aphthous ulcers or larger lesions, with normal mucosa in-between, in the neoterminal ileum (with or without anastomotic lesions)
		i3	Diffuse aphthous ileitis with diffusely inflamed mucosa
		i4	Large ulcers with diffuse mucosal inflammation or nodules or stenosis in the neoterminal ileum

(continued)

Table 6.1 (continued)

Score	Applicability	Variable	Grading
CDEIS	Luminal CD	Deep ulcers	12 if present, 0 if absent
		Superficial ulcers	(6 if present, 0 if absent)
		Surface involved by disease (cm VAS)	0–10 (as the result of visuoanalogic scale transformation representing a complete ileocolonic segment)
		Ulcerated surface (cm VAS)	0–10 (as the result of visuoanalogic scale transformation representing a complete ileocolonic segment)
		Ulcerated stenosis	Quote 3 if ulcerated stenosis anywhere, 0 if not
		Non-ulcerated stenosis	Quote 3 if non-ulcerated stenosis anywhere, 0 if not
SES-CD	Luminal CD	Size of ulcers	0: None 1: Aphthous ulcers ($\varnothing$0.1 to 0.5 cm) 2: Large ulcers ($\varnothing$0.5 to 2 cm) 3: Very large ulcers ($\varnothing$ > 2 cm)
		Ulcerated surface	0: None 1: <10% 2: 10–30% 3: >30%
		Affected surface	0: Unaffected 1: <50% 2: 50–75% 3: >75%
		Presence of narrowing	0: None 1: Single, can be passed 2: Multiple, can be passed 3: Cannot be passed

6.2.1 Mayo Score

The Mayo score is a composite score that includes clinical and endoscopic elements in the assessment of disease activity. The four variables are stool frequency, rectal bleeding, physician's global assessment, and changes in the rectosigmoid mucosa at flexible endoscopy. The endoscopic subsection has a 4-point grading scale for categories ranging from normal to severe disease (0—normal/inactive disease; 1—mild disease: erythema, reduced vascular pattern, mild friability; 2—moderate disease: marked erythema, absent vascular pattern, friability, mucosal erosions; 3—severe disease: spontaneous bleeding, ulceration).

The strengths of the Mayo endoscopic sub-score lie in the frequency of its use in clinical trials, and its ease of use. Its weakness lies in its lack of validation, the lack of differentiation between deep and superficial ulceration and the only focus on the most severely affected segment of the bowel visualized without any indication of the extent or distribution of mucosal inflammation and setting no minimal insertion length [5,

6]. Moreover, this score includes variable degrees of friability in the score of 1 and 2, which results in high inter-observer discrepancy and inconsistent results.

Reasonable concordance ($\kappa = 0.58$; 0.26–0.89) between the Pediatric Ulcerative Colitis Activity Index (PUCAI) and endoscopic Mayo sub-scores was demonstrated in a post hoc analysis of the pediatric trial of infliximab in ulcerative colitis [7].

6.2.2   Ulcerative Colitis Endoscopic Index of Severity (UCEIS)

This index has been developed prospectively and recently validated [8, 9]. From ten initial descriptors, the UCEIS was constructed using regression modelling around three descriptors—vascular pattering, bleeding, and erosions/ulcers. Severity, in terms of UCEIS scores, was compared to a visual analogue scale of overall endoscopic severity. Subsequent validation studies have shown good inter- and intra-observer reliability. Mucosal friability is not included because of the significant inter- and intra-observer variation of this item. UCEIS correlated well with both full and partial Mayo scores, as well as a global rating of endoscopic severity based on a visual analogue scale. Indeed, the UCEIS is currently the most cited tool for assessing the endoscopic severity of UC in adults. Nevertheless, further studies are required to establish thresholds, the clinical relevance of different UCEIS scores, and to explore more deeply its sensitivity-to-change [2, 3]. Interestingly, prior knowledge of clinical data had only a modest effect on UCEIS scores, apart from the description of bleeding at endoscopy.

6.2.3   Ulcerative Colitis Colonoscopic Index of Severity (UCCIS)

This index has been developed prospectively and encompasses assessments of four mucosal variables—vascular pattern, granularity, bleeding/friability, and ulceration in five colonic segments along the entire colon [9–11]. Inter-observer variability was greater in the cecum/ascending colon than in distal segments; bleeding and friability showed only moderate correlation in the descending and sigmoid colon segments. The index correlated well with clinical and laboratory parameters of disease activity. This index has not been validated in multicenter international studies that include nonambulatory patients, and cutoff values for meaningful change, remission, mild, moderate and severe disease activity have yet to be defined.

6.3   Crohn's Disease

6.3.1   Crohn's Disease Endoscopic Index of Severity (CDEIS)

The CDEIS was first developed by the GroupedÉtudeThérapeutique des Affections Inflammatories Digestives (GETAID) [12]. This index scores the presence of superficial or deep ulcers present in each examined segment (rectum, sigmoid and left colon, transverse colon, right colon and ileum). The affected and ulcerated areas are assessed using two visual analogue scales. The scoring sheet for CDEIS is shown in Table 6.1.

The CDEIS is often considered the gold standard for classifying endoscopic disease activity in CD. It is highly reproducible and sensitive to changes in endoscopic mucosal appearance and healing [13]. The CDEIS is the most commonly used endoscopic tool to assess disease activity in clinical trials although there is no agreement or formal validation regarding cutoff values for defining endoscopic response to treatment, endoscopic remission or mucosal healing and no data available on long-term clinical outcomes, especially in children. The main limitation of the CDEIS is its complexity, that requires training and experience to utilize, reserving its use mostly in clinical trials [14].

6.3.2   Simple Endoscopic Score for CD (SES-CD)

The SES-CD score was developed to simplify the CDEIS without losing precision and reproducibility [15]. It was shown to have a close correlation with CDEIS (Spearman's rank order correlation coefficient 0.938, $p < 0.0001$). The most relevant updates were: (1) changes in the definition of ulcers (aphthous, large, and very large ulcers); (2) establishment of a functional definition of narrowing instead of ulcerated or not ulcerated stenosis; (3) change from VAS to 4-modality Likert scales to assess the affected and ulcerated surfaces.

Two major limitations of this score are: (1) the absence of formally validated cutoff values for inactive, mild, moderate, or severe endoscopic activity and (2) the lack of inter-observer agreement.

6.3.3   The Rutgeerts Score

The Rutgeerts score is used for assessing endoscopic activity in the neoterminal ileum after ileocecal resection. Although it has not been fully prospectively validated, the severity of the Rutgeerts score on endoscopy in an asymptomatic patient within 12 months of the ileocolonic resection has been shown to predict the risk of clinical recurrence (low risk with grade 0 or 1; high risk with grade 3 or 4) [16]. A modified Rutgeerts score has not been yet validated (Table 6.1) [17].

6.4   Mucosal Healing

The International Organization for the Study of Inflammatory Bowel Diseases (IOIBD) has recently published a position paper defining the treatment targets and mucosal healing definition.by [18]. For adult patients, mucosal healing has described as the absence of all visible ulcers [18]. This definition is simple to apply in clinical practice, but insensitive to change, and does not allow for a quantification of overall improvement or improvement beyond ulcer healing [19]. For this reason, scoring systems are of critical importance in defining MH in clinical practice [1–3]. Ideally, mucosal healing would mean a SES-CD or CDEIS and a Mayo or UCEIS of 0, but this is not realistic in most cases. Therefore, a SES-CD or CDEIS ≤2 and a Mayo or UCEIS ≤1 have been considered for *endoscopic remission* in CD and UC, respectively [4, 10, 20]. While after surgery in CD, a value of <i2 of Rutgeerts score is considered for endoscopic remission [21].

If mucosal healing or endoscopic remission is not obtained, the treatment efficacy has to be assessed, by defining the *endoscopic response*.

The IOIBD defines *endoscopic response* as a decrease in CDEIS >5 or SES-CD ≥2 for CD, while a decrease in Mayo endoscopic sub-score ≥1 or in UCEIS ≥2 for UC (50). Using relative (rather than absolute) changes, endoscopic response is a decrease of at least 50% from baseline. Indeed, recently, a post hoc analysis of the SONIC trial showed that endoscopic response could be defined as a decrease of at least 50% from baseline [22].

References

1. Dulai PS, Levesque BG, Feagan BG, et al. Assessment of mucosal healing in inflammatory bowel disease: review. Gastrointest Endosc. 2015;82:246–55.
2. Samaan MA, Mosli MH, Sandborn WJ, et al. A systematic review of the measurement of endoscopic healing in ulcerative colitis clinical trials: recommendations and implications for future research. Inflamm Bowel Dis. 2014;20:1465–71.
3. Khanna R, Khanna R, Bouguen G, et al. A systematic review of measurement of endoscopic disease activity and mucosal healing in Crohn's disease: recommendations for clinical trial design. Inflamm Bowel Dis. 2014;20:1850–61.
4. Annese V, Daperno M, Rutter MD, et al. European evidence based consensus for endoscopy in inflammatory bowel disease. J Crohns Colitis. 2013;7:982–1018.
5. Schroeder KW, Tremaine WJ, Ilstrup DM. Coated oral 5-aminosalicylic acid therapy for mildly to moderately active ulcerative colitis. A randomized study. N Engl J Med. 1987;317:1625–9.
6. Mazzuoli S, Guglielmi FW, Antonelli E, et al. Definition and evaluation of mucosal healing in clinical practice. Dig Liver Dis. 2013;45:969–77.
7. Turner D, Griffiths AM, Veerman G, et al. Endoscopic and clinical variables that predict sustained remission in children with ulcerative colitis treated with infliximab. Clin Gastroenterol Hepatol. 2013;11:1460–5.
8. Travis SP, Schnell D, Krzeski P, et al. Developing an instrument to assess the endoscopic severity of ulcerative colitis: the Ulcerative Colitis Endoscopic Index of Severity (UCEIS). Gut. 2012;61:535–42.
9. Samuel S, Bruining DH, Loftus EV Jr, et al. Validation of the ulcerative colitis colonoscopic index of severity and its correlation with disease activity measures. Clin Gastroenterol Hepatol. 2013;11:49–54.
10. Vuitton L, Peyrin-Biroulet L, Colombel JF, et al. Defining endoscopic response and remission in ulcerative colitis clinical trials: an international consensus. Aliment Pharmacol Ther. 2017;45:801–13.
11. Thia KT, Loftus EV Jr, Pardi DS, et al. Measurement of disease activity in ulcerative colitis: interobserver agreement and predictors of severity. Inflamm Bowel Dis. 2011;17:1257–64.
12. Mary JY, Modigliani R. Development and validation of an endoscopic index of the severity for Crohn's disease: a prospective multicentre study. Groupe d'Etudes Therapeutiques des Affections Inflammatoires du Tube Digestif (GETAID). Gut. 1989;30:983–9.

13. Rutgeerts P, Diamond RH, Bala M, et al. Scheduled maintenance treatment with infliximab is superior to episodic treatment for the healing of mucosal ulceration associated with Crohn's disease. Gastrointest Endosc. 2006;63:433–42.
14. Sanborn WJ, et al. A review of activity indices and efficacy endpoints for clinical trials of medical therapy in adults with Crohn's disease. Gastroenterology. 2002;112:512–30.
15. Daperno M, D'Haens G, Van Assche G, et al. Development and validation of a new, simplified endoscopic activity score for Crohn's disease: the SES-CD. Gastrointest Endosc. 2004;60:505–12.
16. Rutgeerts P, Geboes K, Vantrappen G, et al. Natural history of recurrent Crohn's disease at the ileocolonic anastomosis after curative surgery. Gut. 1984;25:665–72.
17. Rutgeerts P, Geboes K, Vantrappen G, et al. Predictability of the postoperative course of Crohn's disease. Gastroenterology. 1990;99:956–63.
18. Peyrin-Biroulet L, Sandborn W, Sands BE, et al. Selecting therapeutic targets in inflammatory bowel disease (STRIDE): determining therapeutic goals for treat-to-target. Am J Gastroenterol. 2015;110:1324–38.
19. Dave M, Loftus EV Jr. Mucosal healing in inflammatory bowel disease-a true paradigm of success? Gastroenterol Hepatol (N Y). 2012;8:29–38.
20. Ruemmele FM, Hyams JS, Otley A, et al. Outcome measures for clinical trials in paediatric IBD: an evidence-based, expert-driven practical statement paper of the paediatric ECCO committee. Gut. 2014;64:438–46.
21. Vuitton L, Marteau P, Sandborn WJ, et al. IOIBD technical review on endoscopic indices for Crohn's disease clinical trials. Gut. 2016;65:1447–55.
22. Ferrante M, et al. Validation of endoscopic activity scores in patients with Crohn's disease based on a post hoc analysis of data from SONIC. Gastroenterology. 2013;145:878–86.

Small-Bowel Endoscopy

7

Paolo Gandullia and Tommaso Bellini

7.1 Introduction

Over the past decade, advances in endoscopic equipment and techniques have allowed diagnostic and therapeutic advancements in the management of small-bowel disorders previously unreachable by standard upper and lower digestive endoscopy [1–4]. The advent of wireless capsule endoscopy (WCE) and balloon-assisted enteroscopy (BAE) between 2000 and 2001 has made the visualization of the entire small-bowel tract easier [5], becoming an attractive diagnostic imaging modality in children for low invasiveness and the absence of ionizing radiation. The inability to obtain tissue samples and to perform intervention has limited the use of WCE [1, 6]. The subsequent advent of BAE has permitted to achieve total small-bowel evaluation, combining both anterograde and retro-grade procedures.

7.2 Technical Features

7.2.1 WCE

The first capsule model was approved by the FDA in 2001, while pediatric use was approved in 2004 and in 2009, respectively, for children between 10 and 18 years old and for all patients over the age ≥ 2 years [7, 8]. The capsule wireless system consists of three components: the endoscopic capsule, the recording system (sensors applied to patient's abdomen and data recorder that is held inside a wearable

P. Gandullia (✉) · T. Bellini
Gastroenterology Unit, G. Gaslini Institute for Maternal and Child Health, IRCCS, Genoa, Italy
e-mail: paologandullia@gaslini.org; paologandullia@ospedale-gaslini.ge.it

© Springer International Publishing AG, part of Springer Nature 2018
L. Dall'Oglio, C. Romano (eds.), *Endoscopy in Pediatric Inflammatory Bowel Disease*,
https://doi.org/10.1007/978-3-319-61249-2_7

belt), and the workstation, where images are downloaded. Real-time visualization software and reconstruction of intestinal transit times are also available. More recently, machine learning algorithms (MLAs) have been proposed to automatically read endoscopic features, and they seem to be as effective as human readers in the diagnosis of small-bowel angioectasias [9].

7.2.2   BAE

Two endoscopes for BAE are currently available: the double balloon enteroscope (DBE—Fujinon Inc. Saitama, Japan), and the single balloon enteroscope (SBE—Olympus, America Inc.). DBE has been first described in 2001, and the first pediatric reports have been reported in 2003 [3, 5, 10]. DBE uses an enteroscope with an inflatable balloon at the distal tip, whereas SBE uses an enteroscopy with no balloon. Both enteroscopes have a length of 200 cm and an outer diameter of 9.4 mm (with operating channel of 2.8 mm); the overtube is 140 cm long and runs on the instrument through a thin film of water that is introduced before performing the procedure to reduce the friction.

7.3   Exam Preparation and Execution

7.3.1   Informed Consent/Refusal [11]

Informed consent in procedural-based medicine is mandatory. It is the tool by which the physician speaks to the patient or patient's surrogate (parents or caregiver in pediatrics) to inform them about a procedure and subsequently obtain legal and ethical permission to perform it. It is recommended that the general indications, methods, risks, benefits, and alternatives to WCE or BAE should be highly explained to the subject and/or appropriate surrogate/caregiver. The benefits of performing WCE or BAE compared with other alternatives should be discussed, and finally the risks of both techniques should be disclosed to the family.

7.3.2   Training/Certification [1, 11]

Universally agreed guidelines for competency in performing advanced endoscopy, such as BAE or WCE, have not been formulated yet. Pediatric gastroenterology training programs do not routinely teach WCE or BAE. There is a wide number of in-person and online training courses endorsed by national or international gastrointestinal societies, whose efficacy has not validated. A minimum of 10–30 WCE are required for trainees to attain competence in WCE. No similar studies about BAEs exist, but some authors suggest a minimum of 20 procedures.

7.3.3 WCE [11–14]

The preparation to perform WCE has not yet been standardized in pediatric population, and there is no strong evidence of which is the best method. The tendency is to perform also an iso-osmolar laxative preparation. The capsule activates just as it is removed from the package and can be swallowed spontaneously by the patient or inserted through endoscopy. Younger children, or patients with difficulty in swallowing, may be trained at home with hard candies, which have approximately the same size as the capsule. A variety of accessories have been used to deliver the capsule endoscope in the stomach or in the small intestine, such as polypectomy snares and nets (both off-label). Only one licensed, dedicated device (US Endoscopy, Mentor, Ohio, USA) is available; that allows the release directly into the duodenum. This procedure requires general anesthesia with airway protection (orotracheal intubation, laryngeal mask).

7.3.4 BAE [2, 4, 6, 10, 13, 15, 16]

Preparation consists of a water diet in the 12–24 h before the procedure and absolute fasting in the previous 4 h; if it has been chosen an anal approach, the preparation for a conventional colonoscopy could be a solution. A general anesthesia with orotracheal intubation is strongly recommended, and it is advisable to use fluoroscopy especially in the early stages of the operator's learning. Both DBE and SBE use an overtube that has a balloon at the distal extremity; by inflating the balloon on the overtube, the small bowel can be reduced and straightened. This straightening facilitates further advancement of the enteroscope, whereas the overtube prevents undesired looping during the procedure. In the DBE, the balloon at the tip of the enteroscope is inflated to anchor the scope in place, whereas the overtube is subsequently advanced before the next reduction. The whole procedure is summarized in Figs. 7.1, 7.2, and 7.3. Choosing which approach to use (anterograde or retrograde) is primarily guided by previous examinations (i.e., entero-MRI), while the absence of indications or lesion locations may suggest to start with an oral approach.

7.4   Indications

WCE and BAE share most of all indications but there may be some difference [10]. Main indications for both techniques in pediatric age is known or suspected IBD.

Conventional upper and lower intestinal endoscopy usually allows a definite diagnosis of IBD, and both WCE and BAE have a limited role in the initial evaluation of patients with known or suspected CD [10, 15]. WCE is indicated, if needed, as first-line enteroscopic tool for small-bowel evaluation and meets several indications: differential diagnosis between ulcerative colitis (UC), CD and unclassified IBD (IBDU); differential diagnosis with other pathological conditions, such as polyps, Meckel diverticulum, intestinal duplications, angiodysplasias, and other

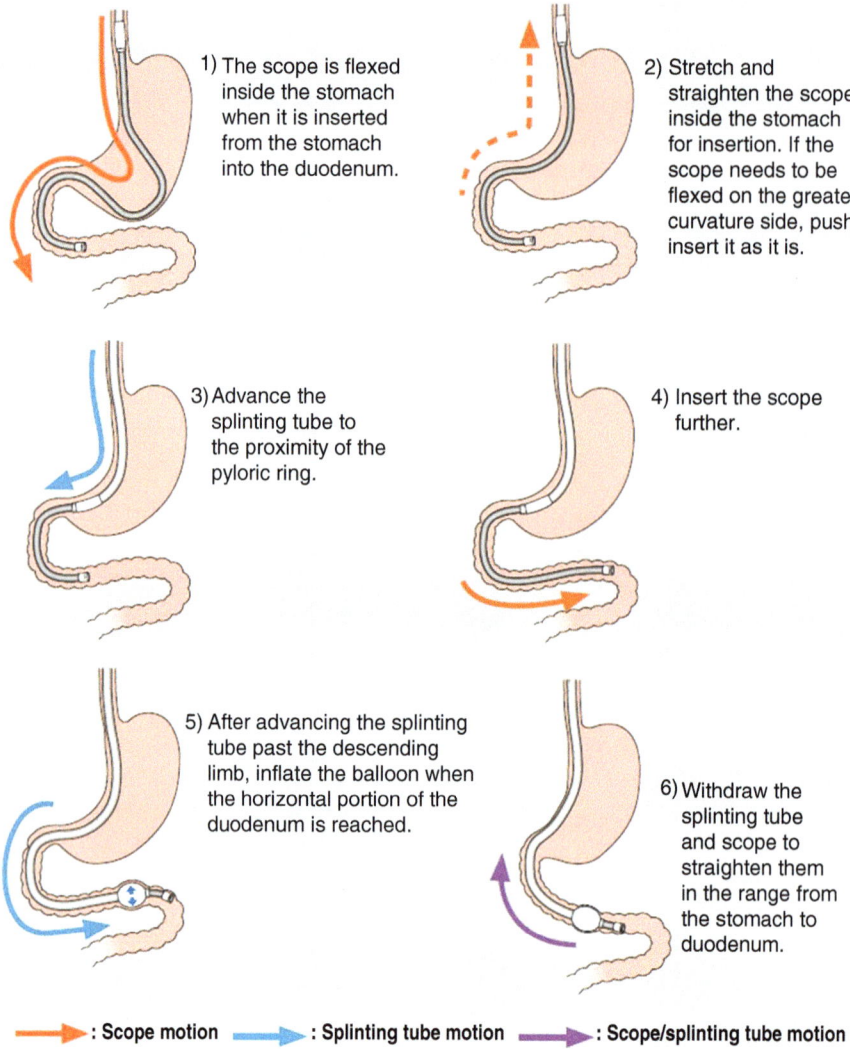

1) The scope is flexed inside the stomach when it is inserted from the stomach into the duodenum.

2) Stretch and straighten the scope inside the stomach for insertion. If the scope needs to be flexed on the greater curvature side, push insert it as it is.

3) Advance the splinting tube to the proximity of the pyloric ring.

4) Insert the scope further.

5) After advancing the splinting tube past the descending limb, inflate the balloon when the horizontal portion of the duodenum is reached.

6) Withdraw the splinting tube and scope to straighten them in the range from the stomach to duodenum.

→ : Scope motion   → : Splinting tube motion   → : Scope/splinting tube motion

Fig. 7.1 Balloon-assisted enteroscopy passing through the stomach and duodenum

vascular malformations; staging of suspected CD with a normal traditional endoscopy; in known CD with unexplained signs or symptoms; surveillance of possible surgical complications (i.e., anastomotic ulcers); monitoring mucosal healing [3, 5, 17–19]. BAE shares with WCE the indications mentioned above; it is also indicated to perform biopsy in case of lesions identified with the WCE. If entero-MRI has already evidenced stenosis/strictures or lesions that deserves histological characterization or a therapeutic intervention (stopping a bleeding, CD-related stenosis/strictures dilation, removal of retained capsule), BAE is of first choice, avoiding the

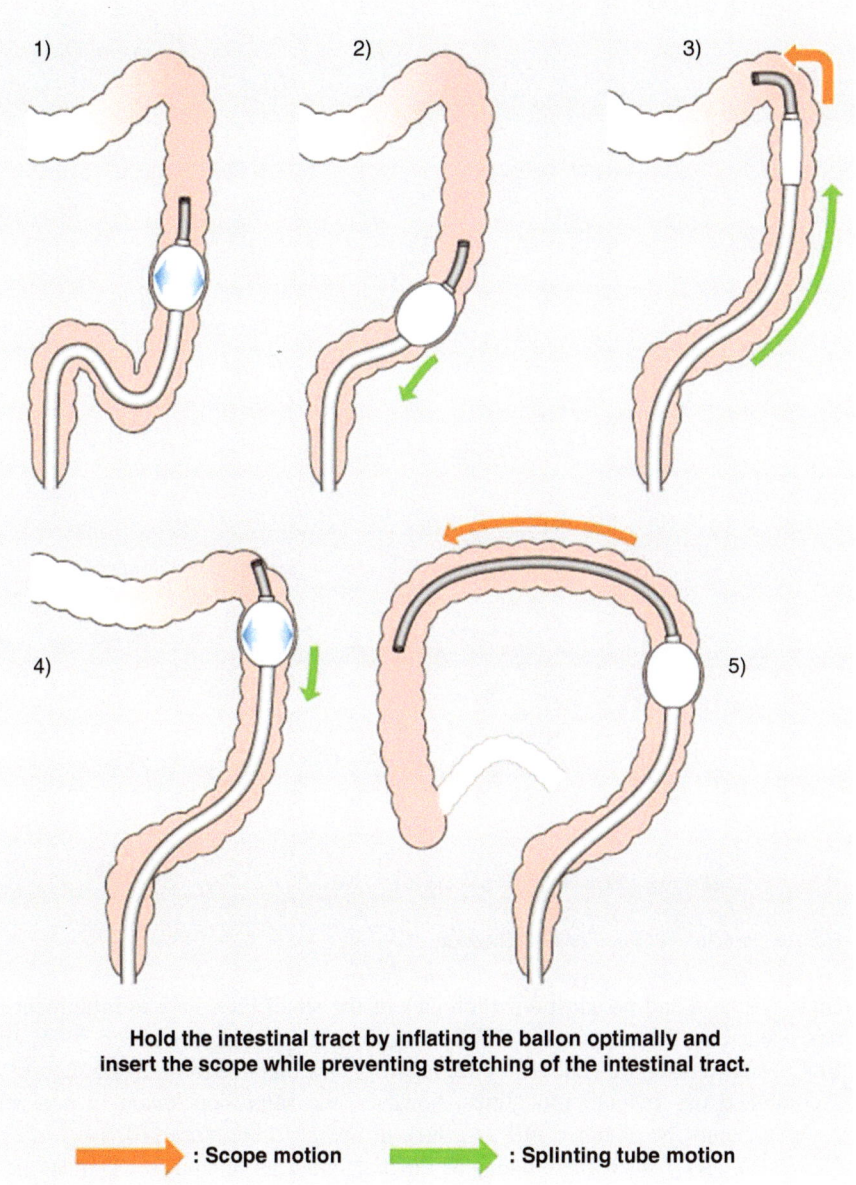

1)

2)

3)

4)

5)

**Hold the intestinal tract by inflating the ballon optimally and
insert the scope while preventing stretching of the intestinal tract.**

➡ : Scope motion   ➡ : Splinting tube motion

Fig. 7.2 Balloon-assisted enteroscopy passing through the colon

WCE [4, 5, 10, 20]. A proposed diagnostic-therapeutic algorithm for CD is reported in Fig. 7.4.

OGIB is defined as a bleeding of unknown origin that persists or recurs, after negative initial evaluation using bidirectional endoscopy and small-bowel imaging. Incidence is low in pediatric age presents a lower incidence because acquired

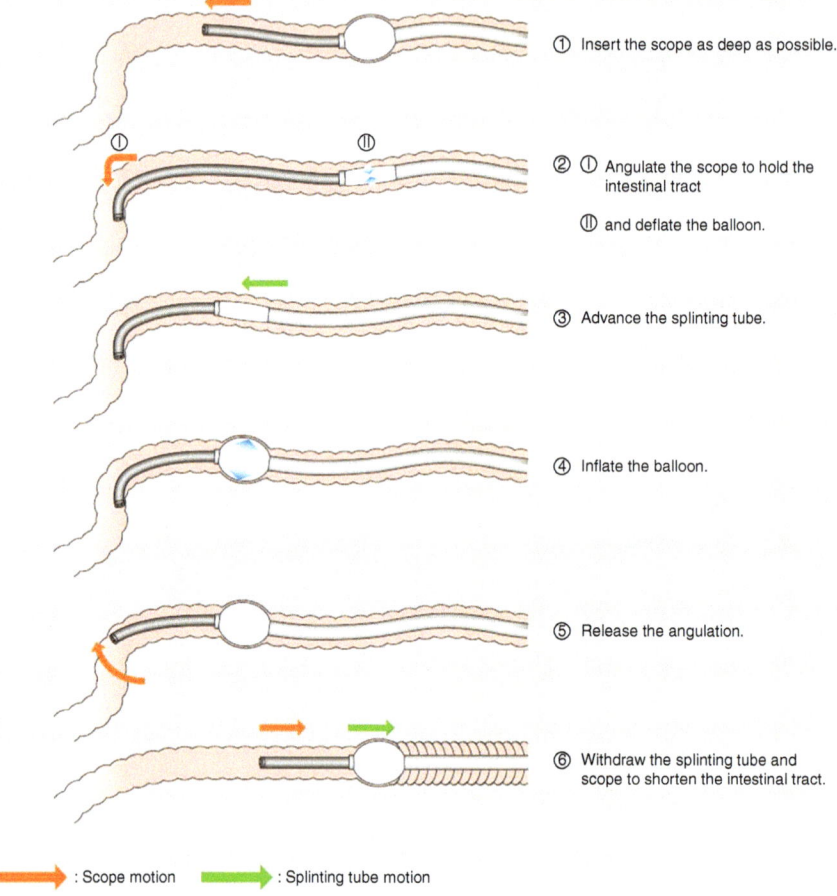

① Insert the scope as deep as possible.

② ① Angulate the scope to hold the intestinal tract

   ① and deflate the balloon.

③ Advance the splinting tube.

④ Inflate the balloon.

⑤ Release the angulation.

⑥ Withdraw the splinting tube and scope to shorten the intestinal tract.

➡ : Scope motion   ➡ : Splinting tube motion

Fig. 7.3 Principles of insertion and retraction

angiodysplasia and neoplastic pathologies of the small intestine are infrequent in this age group. In adults with OGIB, diagnostic comparison between WCE and BAE revealed no significant difference regarding the diagnostic yield and supported a combined use of both modalities; however, the same conclusion in pediatric patients cannot be obtained due to a lack in pediatric literature [10, 14, 17, 21]. OGIB and unexplained anemia may be the first symptom of an ileal CD or surgical complications.

7.5   Contraindications

Patient selection must be rigid: patients should undergo to high and low endoscopic examination and imaging of the small intestine to exclude digestive tract lesions that could represent a contraindication (see below) [6, 11, 14].

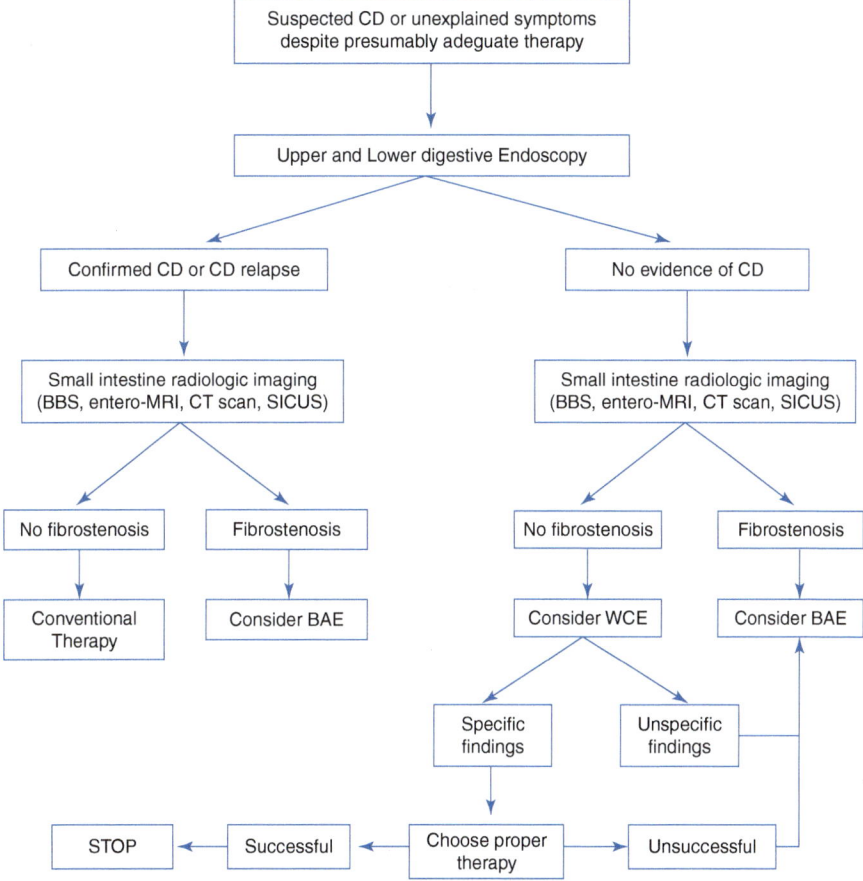

Fig. 7.4 A proposed algorithm for the evaluation of suspected or relapsed CD (revised from [1, 13]). *BBS* barium series studies, *entero-MRI* entero magnetic resonance, *CT scan* abdominal contrast enhanced computed tomography, *SICUS* small-intestine contrast ultrasound, *WCE* wireless capsule endoscopy, *BAE* balloon-assisted enteroscopy

7.5.1 WCE [3, 7, 8, 11, 12, 14, 22]

Relative contraindications of WCE include any condition in which obstruction, strictures, or fistulae are suspected, which could cause WCE retention, and are listed in Table 7.1. In adults, a patency capsule (PC) is swallowed before the formal WCE study, in order to establish luminal patency and minimize the risk of capsule retention; the PC is not equipped with a camera but is radiologically identifiable and it is absorbable in 36–48 h if not expelled. Younger children cannot swallow the PC and sedation only for endoscopic placement of the PC is not recommended: it is suggested to perform a small-bowel anatomical study (BSS, CT scan, or entero-MRI) to help in predicting the risk of capsule retention, especially in high-risk patients. Normal imaging, however, does not obviate the risk of capsule retention.

Table 7.1 Contraindications for BAE and WCE in pediatric age

Balloon-assisted enteroscopy		
Absolute	Related	Wireless capsule endoscopy
– Intestinal perforation	– Age or weight	– Bowel obstruction
– Peritonitis	– Thrombocytopenia or	(Suspected or known)
– Septic state	coagulopathy	– Bowel strictures
– Hemodynamic	– Severe neutropenia	– Bowel fistula
instability	– Recent digestive surgery or	– Age or weight
	adhesions	– Allergy to materials
	– Intestinal occlusion	– Presence of pacemaker or other
	– Vascular aneurysms	electromagnetic device

There is no weight or age limit to perform WCE in children, even in <2 years old WCE is off-label. With the endoscopy-assisted placement of the WCE, studies have been successfully performed in children as young as 10 months and 7.9 kg, but the size of patient and the size of oral and pharyngeal tissues may pose a limitation; thus, caution should be approached when placing WCE in such small children. Other studies have proposed 11.5 kg as lower weight and 18 months as lower age to perform WCE.

7.5.2 BAE [6, 13]

Absolute contraindications are intestinal perforation or peritonitis, a septic state and/or an hemodynamic instability. Related contraindications are listed in Table 7.1.

It has not been well established which are the minimum weight and/or age to perform the exam; to date, BAE seems feasible in children as young as 3 years and as small as 13 kg, but there are only few, mostly retrospective, available data on a small number of patients. Moreover, appropriately sized endoscopes for even smaller sized patients are not available yet.

7.6 Complications

7.6.1 WCE [2, 3, 6–8, 13, 14, 22, 23]

WCE is generally a well-tolerated and safe procedure. Minor complications include skin or mucosal irritation, vomiting, pain, sore throat, missed lesion, or equipment malfunction. The most serious complication that may occur during the examination is the capsule retention, which has been defined as a WCE remaining in the intestinal lumen for 2 or more weeks or as a WCE that has required directed therapy to aid its passage. Unless a patient is symptomatic, the first clue of a retained capsule is the discovery of an incomplete study, in which the capsule does not reach the cecum at the conclusion of the study. In cases where the capsule retention in the intestinal lumen occurs for more than 15 days or becomes symptomatic, a surgical or endoscopic removal is mandatory, even if it has been described a spontaneous capsule evacuation after 3 months of retention.

7.6.2   BAE [2, 3, 6, 17, 24]

The lower number of complications with BAE is mainly due to the few pediatric cases; two recent pediatric studies demonstrate that SBE is safe and well tolerated. Common complications include perforation, pancreatitis, and bleeding, and are noticeably more frequent in patients with adherences, altered intestinal anatomy or repeated procedures (i.e., in polyposis syndromes). Minor complications, such as self-limited abdominal pain and/or distension, sore throat, nausea, have the same frequency than with conventional gastroscopy and colonoscopy examinations.

7.7   Limitations

The main WCE limitations are the inability to wash and aspirate secretions in the lumen, and the inability to obtain biopsies; the latest guidelines suggest that CD diagnosis should never be made only on the results of a WCE test [18]. Principal limitation in BAE is due to the operator experience; hence, it is important to emphasize that these procedures should be performed in third-level pediatric centers by highly specialized and qualified personnel [1].

Conclusions

WCE and BAE are newer endoscopic modalities that have improved both diagnosis and treatment of small-bowel pathology in pediatric patients [7]. WCE is a very useful approach to children presenting symptoms suggesting IBD, as a third-stage examination after conventional upper and lower GI endoscopy [9, 10]. In presence of small-bowel stenosis on radiologic imaging, BAE may allow both diagnosis and therapeutic treatment and may avoid a surgical intervention. BAE is more invasive and less safe than WCE. It shows therapeutic advantages in IBD, such as the possibility to place tattoos, perform hemostasis, dilate CD strictures and stenosis, and remove foreign bodies (including retained capsules) [15]. The diagnostic capability of the two BAE instruments (DBE, SBE) seems to overlap, so the choice is guided mainly by operator experience. WCE use is suggested as a first-line study in patients with a negative previous workup for CD (including upper and lower endoscopy and small-bowel imaging tests), and then BAE, if needed (Fig. 7.4). BAE could be used as a first-line technique if a pathological study has showed a WCE contraindication or if an endoscopic therapy is needed (i.e., strictures dilatation, hemostasis) [1, 13, 18, 25]. WCE and DBE may be performed in tandem, with initial WCE findings directing the choice of antegrade versus retrograde DBE approach. Recent results show how the two techniques combined can be complementary and fill the limits of each other.

Future studies, comparing WCE and BAE and defining their precise role, would clarify the diagnostic and therapeutic algorithms for management of IBD and other small-bowel diseases in children.

References

1. Steiner SJ. Deeper and deeper into the pediatric small bowel. Gastrointest Endosc. 2012;75(1):95–7. https://doi.org/10.1016/j.gie.2011.08.048.
2. Barth BA, Channabasappa N. Single-balloon enteroscopy in children: initial experience at a pediatric center. J Pediatr Gastroenterol Nutr. 2010;51(5):680–4. https://doi.org/10.1097/MPG.0b013e3181e85b3d.
3. deRidder L, Tabbers MM, Escher JC. Small bowel endoscopy in children. Best Pract Res Clin Gastroenterol. 2012;26(3):337–45. https://doi.org/10.1016/j.bpg.2012.02.001.
4. Chen WG, Shan GD, Zhang H, Yang M, L L, Yue M, et al. Double-balloon enteroscopy in small bowel diseases: eight years single-center experience in China. Medicine (Baltimore). 2016;95(42):e5104.
5. ASGE Standards of Practice Committee, Khashab MA, Pasha SF, Muthusamy VR, Acosta RD, Bruining DH, Chandrasekhara V, et al. The role of deep enteroscopy in the management of small-bowel disorders. Gastrointest Endosc. 2015;82(4):600–7. https://doi.org/10.1016/j.gie.2015.06.046.
6. Yokoyama K, Yano T, Kumagai H, Mizuta K, Ono S, Imagawa T, et al. Double-balloon enteroscopy for pediatric patients: evaluation of safety and efficacy in 257 cases. J Pediatr Gastroenterol Nutr. 2016;63(1):34–40. https://doi.org/10.1097/MPG.0000000000001048.
7. Cohen SA, Ephrath H, Lewis JD, Klevens A, Bergwerk A, Liu S, et al. Pediatric capsule endoscopy: review of the small bowel and patency capsules. J Pediatr Gastroenterol Nutr. 2012;54(3):409–13. https://doi.org/10.1097/MPG.0b013e31822c81fd.
8. Mishkin DS, Chuttani R, Croffie J, Disario J, Liu J, Shah R, et al. ASGE Technology Status Evaluation Report: wireless capsule endoscopy. Gastrointest Endosc. 2006;63(4):539–45.
9. Koulaouzidis A, Iakovidis DK, Yung DE, Rondonotti E, Kopylov U, Plevris JN, et al. KID Project: an internet-based digital video atlas of capsule endoscopy for research purposes. Endosc Int Open. 2017;5(6):E477–83. https://doi.org/10.1055/s-0043-105488.
10. Di Nardo G, Oliva S, Aloi M, Rossi P, Casciani E, Masselli G, et al. Usefulness of single-balloon enteroscopy in pediatric Crohn's disease. Gastrointest Endosc. 2012;75(1):80–6. https://doi.org/10.1016/j.gie.2011.06.021.
11. Friedlander JA, Liu QY, Sahn B, Kooros K, Walsh CM, Kramer RE, et al. NASPGHAN Capsule Endoscopy Clinical Report. J Pediatr Gastroenterol Nutr. 2017;64(3):485–94. https://doi.org/10.1097/MPG.0000000000001413.
12. de'Angelis GL, Fornaroli F, de'Angelis N, Magiteri B, Bizzarri B. Wireless capsule endoscopy for pediatric small-bowel diseases. Am J Gastroenterol. 2007;102(8):1749–57.
13. Di Nardo G, de Ridder L, Oliva S, Casciani E, Escher JC, Cucchiara S. Enteroscopy in paediatric Crohn's disease. Dig Liver Dis. 2013;45(5):351–5. https://doi.org/10.1016/j.dld.2012.07.020.
14. Danialifar TF, Naon H, Liu QY. Comparison of diagnostic accuracy and concordance of video capsule endoscopy and double balloon enteroscopy in children. J Pediatr Gastroenterol Nutr. 2016;62(6):824–7. https://doi.org/10.1097/MPG.0000000000001066.
15. deRidder L, Mensink PB, Lequin MH, Aktas H, de Krijger RR, van der Woude CJ, et al. Single-balloon enteroscopy, magnetic resonance enterography, and abdominal US useful for evaluation of small-bowel disease in children with (suspected) Crohn's disease. Gastrointest Endosc. 2012;75(1):87–94. https://doi.org/10.1016/j.gie.2011.07.036.
16. Tringali A, Thomson M, Dumonceau JM, Tavares M, Tabbers MM, Furlano R, et al. Pediatric gastrointestinal endoscopy: European Society of Gastrointestinal Endoscopy (ESGE) and European Society for Paediatric Gastroenterology Hepatology and Nutrition (ESPGHAN) guideline executive summary. Endoscopy. 2017;49(1):83–91. https://doi.org/10.1055/s-0042-111002.
17. Rahman A, Ross A, Leighton JA, Schembre D, Gerson L, Lo SK, et al. Double-balloon enteroscopy in Crohn's disease: findings and impact on management in a multicenter retrospective study. Gastrointest Endosc. 2015;82(1):102–7. https://doi.org/10.1016/j.gie.2014.12.039.

18. Di Nardo G, Oliva S, Ferrari F, Riccioni ME, Staiano A, Lombardi G, et al. Usefulness of wireless capsule endoscopy in paediatric inflammatory bowel disease. Dig Liver Dis. 2011;43(3):220–4. https://doi.org/10.1016/j.dld.2010.10.004.

19. Levine A, Koletzko S, Turner D, Escher JC, Cucchiara S, de Ridder L, et al. ESPGHAN revised porto criteria for the diagnosis of inflammatory bowel disease in children and adolescents. J Pediatr Gastroenterol Nutr. 2014;58(6):795–806. https://doi.org/10.1097/MPG.0000000000000239.

20. Uchida K, Yoshiyama S, Inoue M, Koike Y, Yasuda H, Fujikawa H, et al. Double balloon enteroscopy for pediatric inflammatory bowel disease. Pediatr Int. 2012;54(6):806–9. https://doi.org/10.1111/j.1442-200X.2012.03661.x.

21. Shen R, Sun B, Gong B, Zhang S, Cheng S. Double-balloon enteroscopy in the evaluation of small bowel disorders in pediatric patients. Dig Endosc. 2012;24(2):87–92. https://doi.org/10.1111/j.1443-1661.2011.01175.x; Epub 2011 Jul 13.

22. Jensen MK, Tipnis NA, Bajorunaite R, Sheth MK, Sato TT, Noel RJ. Capsule endoscopy performed across the pediatric age range: indications, incomplete studies, and utility in management of inflammatory bowel disease. Gastrointest Endosc. 2010;72(1):95–102. https://doi.org/10.1016/j.gie.2010.01.016.

23. Herle K, Jehangir S. Retained wireless capsule endoscope in a girl with suspected Crohn's disease. APSP J Case Rep. 2016;7(4):27. https://doi.org/10.21699/ajcr.v7i4.466.

24. Moreels TG, Di Nardo G. The next novelty in pediatric endoscopy: enteroscopy. J Pediatr Gastroenterol Nutr. 2014;58(2):141–2. https://doi.org/10.1097/MPG.0000000000000193.

25. Oliva S, Pennazio M, Cohen SA, Aloi M, Barabino A, Hassan C, et al. Capsule endoscopy followed by single balloon enteroscopy in children with obscure gastrointestinal bleeding: a combined approach. Dig Liver Dis. 2015;47(2):125–30. https://doi.org/10.1016/j.dld.2014.09.001.

Operative Endoscopy in Pediatric Inflammatory Bowel Disease

8

Erminia Romeo, Filippo Torroni, and Luigi Dall'Oglio

8.1 Dilation Technique

Catheters used for gastrointestinal strictures dilation are: an over-the-wire balloon catheter and a through-the-scope (TTS) balloon catheter, usually preferred. The length of the balloons for inflation is about 5 cm; therefore, strictures 5 cm or longer are considered unsuitable for EBD, but sometimes a step-by-step dilation can be performed [1]. Intestinal strictures with deep ulcers and fistulous complications are contraindication for EBD. The dilation procedure is performed under X-ray guidance for monitoring the inflated balloon [2]. In pediatric patients, all operative procedures are performed under general anesthesia in operative room. The maximum dilation diameter ranges among 18 mm, 20 mm, and 25 mm, generally 18–20 mm is the most common. Successful dilation is considered as disappearance of stenotic symptoms or the ability to pass a scope as a technical response (79–100%) [1] (Figs. 8.1 and 8.2).

Perforation and bleeding are the major concerns during the procedure. The rate of perforation is nearby <10%, and it requires emergent surgery [3].

EBD for Crohn's strictures may be a good therapeutic option at least for the temporary relief of stenotic symptoms. The relapse rate of obstructive symptoms after EBD ranges from 24 to 79% [4]. In patients with recurrence of symptoms, redilation or surgical intervention should be performed. According to a meta-analysis that summarized 25 studies, including 1089 patients and 2664 dilations, the proportion of patients who required further dilation at 1, 2, and 5 years of follow-up was 31.6%, 25.9%, and 1.7%, respectively [5]. The surgical intervention rate is 27% [4].

E. Romeo (✉) · F. Torroni · L. Dall'Oglio
Digestive Surgery and Endoscopy Unit, Bambino Gesù Children's Hospital, Rome, Italy
e-mail: erminia.romeo@opbg.net; Luigi.dalloglio@opbg.net

© Springer International Publishing AG, part of Springer Nature 2018
L. Dall'Oglio, C. Romano (eds.), *Endoscopy in Pediatric Inflammatory Bowel Disease*,
https://doi.org/10.1007/978-3-319-61249-2_8

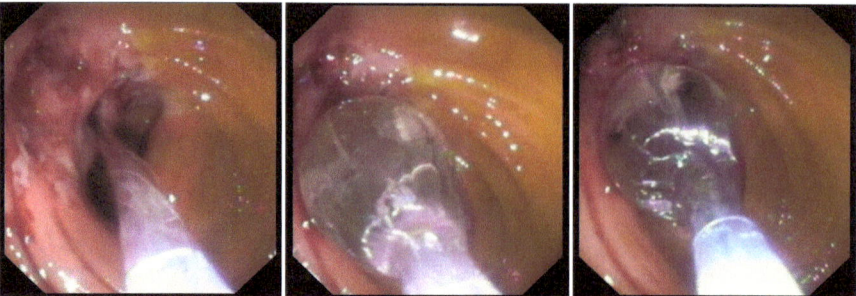

Fig. 8.1 Ileo-cecal valve dilation. TTS catheter. Digestive Surgery and Endoscopy Unit. Bambino Gesù Children's Hospital, Italy

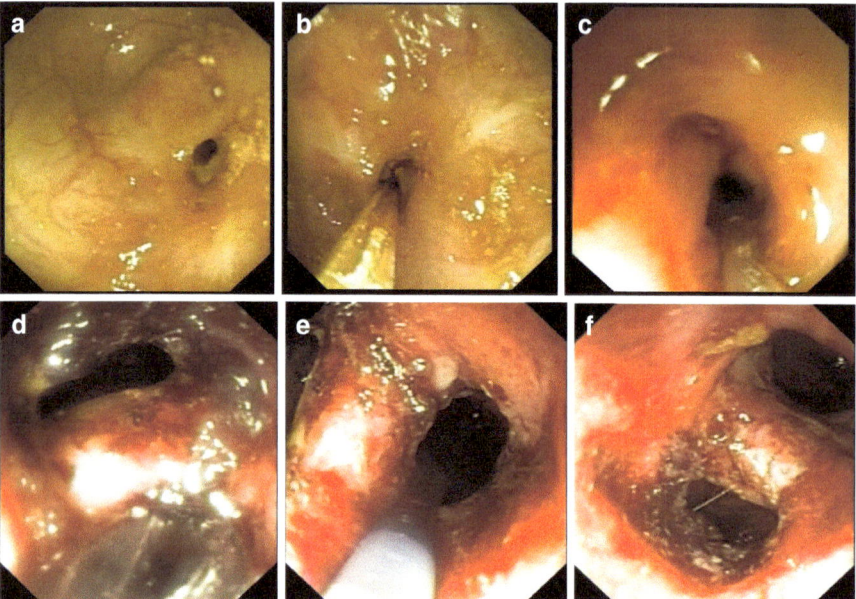

Fig. 8.2 (**a**) Cecal stricture; (**b**) over-the-wire catheter dilation; (**c**) after dilation; (**d**) ileo-cecal valve stricture dilation with TTS catheter; (**e**) after dilation; (**f**) ileo-cecal valve dilation and cecal dilation. Digestive Surgery and Endoscopy Unit. Bambino Gesù Children's Hospital, Italy

8.2 Factors Associated with Favorable Outcomes

Many factors are involved in determining endoscopic dilation outcomes.

Primary strictures were significantly associated with decreased surgery-free intervals in the long term; [6]; EBD in anastomotic strictures appear to be more effective and with a good outcome in the long-term follow-up [6].

The length of the strictures is a determinant of the outcome of balloon dilation; stricture length >4 cm is associated with a poor outcome [4].

Post-dilation pharmacotherapy with steroids or immunomodulators has not yielded significant changes in the efficacy of dilation [4].

The use of self-expandable metal stents in selected patients, especially those with benign refractory strictures, was found to be safe and effective in a small case series of five patients, and this can improve the efficacy of EBD. However, there is a risk of stent migration, and large prospective trials are still lacking in this area [7].

8.3   EBD Using BAE for Small Bowel Strictures

EBD using BAE for small bowel strictures is almost the same as EBD for colorectal and ileo-colonic strictures in terms of procedure and technique; catheters are the same used with a standard colonoscope.

There are some technical difficulties, compared to EBD performed with a conventional colonoscope. According to published studies, maximum dilation diameter for strictures of the small intestine varied from 15 to 20 mm, smaller than those of colorectal and ileo-colonic strictures. Nonetheless, the reported technical success rate (such as 72–100%) and cumulative redilation-free rate (such as 64% and 47%, respectively, at 2 and 3 years) are similar to those of EBD for colorectal and ileo-colonic strictures [1].

Therefore, the need for frequent redilation seems to be an issue with EBD regardless of the target stricture site. According to a recent study published by Sunada et al., the cumulative surgery-free rate after initial EBD for small bowel strictures in CD was 87.3% at 1 year and 78.1% at 3 years [2].

The tendency for CD patients to have multiple small bowel strictures is one of the limitations of EBD using BAE.

In some cases, BAE is used for retrieving capsule endoscopy impacted in small bowel stricture, with standard foreign body roth net (Fig. 8.3).

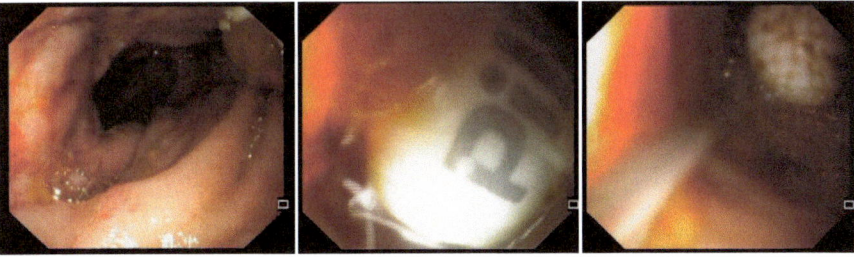

Fig. 8.3 Small bowel sub-stenosis; capsule impaction; capsule retrieval. Digestive Surgery and Endoscopy Unit. Bambino Gesù Children's Hospital, Italy

Conclusions

Intestinal strictures are still a major cause of surgery in CD. Since frequent intestinal resection often results in short bowel syndrome and can decrease the quality of life, EBD can help avoid surgery. EBD with a conventional colonoscope for Crohn's strictures of the colon and ileo-colonic anastomosis, self-expanding stent, EBD with a balloon-assisted enteroscope seems to be effective and safe.

References

1. Despott EJ, Gupta A, Burling D, et al. Effective dilation of small bowel strictures by double-balloon enteroscopy in patients with symptomatic Crohn's disease. Gastrointest Endosc. 2009;70:1030–6.
2. Sunada K, Shinozaki S, Nagayama M, et al. Long-term outcomes in patients with small intestinal strictures secondary to Crohn's disease after double-balloon endoscopy-assisted balloon dilation. Inflamm Bowel Dis. 2016;22:380–6.
3. Hirai F. Current status of endoscopic balloon dilation for Crohn's disease. Intest Res. 2017;15:166–73.
4. Navaneethan U, Lourdusamy V, Njei B, et al. Endoscopic balloon dilation in the management of strictures in Crohn's disease: a systematic review and meta-analysis of non-randomized trials. Surg Endosc. 2016;30:5434–43.
5. Morar PS, Faiz O, Warusavitarne J, et al. Systematic review with meta-analysis: endoscopic balloon dilatation for Crohn's disease strictures. Aliment Pharmacol Ther. 2015;42:1137–48.
6. Mueller T, Rieder B, Bechtner G, et al. The response of Crohn's strictures to endoscopic balloon dilation. Aliment Pharmacol Ther. 2010;31:634–9.
7. Levine RA, Wasvary H, Kadro O. Endoprosthetic management of refractory ileocolonic anastomotic strictures after resection for Crohn's disease: report of nine-year follow-up and review of the literature. Inflamm Bowel Dis. 2012;18(3):506–12.

Cancer and Dysplasia Surveillance

9

Gian Luigi de'Angelis, Federica Gaiani,
and Nicola de'Angelis

9.1 Introduction

The increased risk of cancer in IBD patients is object of a worldwide consensus of the literature, both for patients affected by UC and for patients affected by CD.

Therefore, the theme of cancer surveillance has become of growing importance in recent decades, in terms of early diagnosis, understanding of the mechanisms for carcinogenesis, and awareness of the risk factors concerning this particular group of patients, including mucosal inflammation and long-term immunosuppression.

From an epidemiologic point of view, cancerous lesions usually develop in the adult age, but the early optimization of the management is of paramount importance for the long course of the disease, starting from the pediatric age.

9.2 Overall Risk of Cancer

With respect to the basic risk of developing specific cancers, pathogenesis and epidemiology, literature data are conflicting. In adult population, a Finnish study reported that UC patients were found to have an increased risk of colon, rectal, biliary tract, and thyroid cancers, and the risk of colorectal cancer (CRC) was highest among the youngest UC patients. CD patients had a significantly increased risk for cancers of the small intestine, anus, and biliary tract, and also for myeloma. The risk of basal cell skin cancer was also increased in IBD [1]. On the contrary, data from

G. L. de'Angelis (✉) · F. Gaiani
Gastroenterology and Endoscopy Unit, Azienda Ospedaliero-Universitaria,
University Hospital of Parma, Parma, Italy
e-mail: gianluigi.deangelis@unipr.it; federica.gaiani@studenti.unipr.it

N. de'Angelis
Department of Digestive, Hepatobiliary Surgery and Liver Transplantation, Henri Mondor
University Hospital, AP-HP, Université Paris Est – UPEC, Créteil, France

© Springer International Publishing AG, part of Springer Nature 2018
L. Dall'Oglio, C. Romano (eds.), *Endoscopy in Pediatric Inflammatory Bowel Disease*,
https://doi.org/10.1007/978-3-319-61249-2_9

Denmark indicated that only CD patients had an increased risk of developing malignancies overall, such as small bowel cancer, lung cancer, or non-Hodgkin lymphoma (NHL), while the general risk for developing cancer in UC patients was not increased [2, 3]. Other correlations between IBD and malignancies have been made with regard to specific immunosuppressors and malignancies, such as thiopurines and lymphoma (especially NHL) [4, 5].

The data on cancer risk of IBD pediatric patients are lacking [6]. One pediatric French population-based study estimated the risk of cancer in patients with childhood-onset CD (median age at diagnosis 14.6 years; median follow-up 11.4 years), and found a non-significant 2.5-fold increase compared with the background population [7]. Similar results were found by a more recent Danish study, in which the overall risk of cancer in a population diagnosed at the age of 19 years or less, was of 2.17-fold increased, compared with non-IBD population [6].

The theme of cancer surveillance in IBD can be divided into cancer and dysplastic lesions of the gastrointestinal tract, extraintestinal malignancies, and predisposition to cancer due to immunosuppressive drugs.

9.3   Cancer and Dysplastic Lesions of the Gastrointestinal Tract

IBD are well-recognized risk factors for the development of colorectal and small bowel cancer.

This assumption is confirmed by numerous literature data: for example, among Indian population, characterized by a low incidence of sporadic CRC, the risk of colorectal cancer (CRC) in patients with UC is high and similar to that in Western countries [8].

In particular, UC and colic CD are risk factors for CRC, which is specifically called colitis-associated colorectal cancer (CAC), while ileal CD has to be surveilled with regard to small bowel cancer (SBA).

9.3.1   Epidemiology

Accordingly with several epidemiological studies, IBD patients have a 2.2 times higher risk of developing CRC compared with the general population [9].

Studies quantifying the increased risk of CRC in patients with IBD have generated variable results reflecting differences in country of origin, study population, and disease duration [10].

An updated meta-analysis of population-based cohort studies has quantified the incidence of CRC among patients with IBD to be 1%, 2%, and 5% after 10, 20, and >20 years of disease duration [11]. Another large meta-analysis assessing CRC risk in patients with IBD showed a risk of 2% at 10 years after UC diagnosis, 8% at 20 years, and 18% at 30 years after colitis onset [8, 12].

Taken together, CAC remains an important consequence of long-standing IBD with an estimated incidence of approximately 5% after 20 years of disease duration [13].

The risk of cancer-related death is 1.9 times greater in patients with UC or CD disease than those without IBD [9].

Important clinical differences exist between CAC and sporadic CRC in the general population:

- CAC is more common among young patients both in case of UC and CD (average age of 50–60 years in IBD compared with 65–75 years for sporadic CRC in the general population) [14]
- CAC is more likely to be found in the proximal colon (51.5%) compared to sporadic CRC (36.4%), especially in the presence of primary sclerosing cholangitis (PSC) [15]
- CAC is more commonly synchronous (15–20% of CAC compared with 3–5% of sporadic CRC)
- CAC is difficult to detect using a barium enema or even by colonoscopy because of its widespread nature
- CAC is characterized by higher proportions of morphologically superficial type lesions and invasive type lesions compared to sporadic CRC
- CAC has an increased frequency of mucinous or signet ring cell histology
- underlying genetic alterations are different [12, 16, 17]

The data on cancer risk in patients with IBD diagnosed in childhood are sparse and focused on the overall risk of cancer rather than on the risk of development of CAC [6]. Among the few studies regarding the risk of CAC, the national cohort from Denmark (1979–2008) found the highest relative risk (RR) of CRC among patients diagnosed less than or equal to 19 years of age compared with the background population (RR 2.35, 95% Confidence Interval (CI): 0.33–16.7) and within the CD cohort (RR 3.66, 95% CI: 0.49–27.6) [2, 6].

Regarding the evolution of the epidemiology of CACs over the years, the incidence rate seems to be lower. This result might be attributed to the improvement of therapies for patients with IBD and to the advent of surveillance colonoscopy programs with early colectomy [14, 18].

Conservative proctocolectomy with ileal pouch-anal anastomosis (IPAA) has become the intervention of choice for severe UC requiring surgery. Although the risk for neoplasia in patients with UC and IPAA is low, it is not negligible.

In a series of 3203 IBD patients who underwent restorative proctocolectomy with IPAA, the cumulative incidences of pouch neoplasia at 5, 10, 15, 20, and 25 years were 0.9%, 1.3%, 1.9%, 4.2%, and 5.1%, respectively. Of these patients, 38 (1.19%) had pouch neoplasia (adenocarcinoma of the pouch and/or Anal Transition Zone (ATZ) in 11 cases [0.36%], pouch lymphoma in 1 [0.03%], squamous cell cancer of the ATZ in 3, and dysplasia in 23 [0.72%]); patients who had undergone mucosectomy had risk too [19]. In a systematic review of 23 observational studies and case series including 2040 patients, the pooled prevalence of confirmed dysplasia involving the pouch, ATZ, or rectal cuff after restorative proctocolectomy for UC was 1.13% (range 0–18.75) [20].

Although specific risk factors for the development are recognized (See paragraph "Risk factors"), accordingly with a retrospective analysis conducted in 2009, post-IPAA cancer can occur:

– after mucosectomy or stapled anastomosis
– after IPAAs performed for UC alone or for UC with neoplasia
– regardless of whether the initial cancer or dysplasia involved the rectum

The risk of small bowel adenocarcinoma is markedly increased in CD, compared to general population, and it has been estimated to range from 6 to 320 [21].

The pathogenesis of SBA in CD is poorly defined, although the regional distribution of Crohn-related SBA which tends to follow the distribution of the disease and the correlation with long-standing active disease seem to attribute to inflammation a crucial pathogenic role [21, 22].

Cancer arising at the site of a chronic perianal fistula is extremely rare in patients with CD. A study conducted along 10 years of observation of CD patients presenting perianal fistulas suggests that carcinoma occurs in <1% of patients [23]. The rarity of this condition limits the ability to establish epidemiological data or any standard protocol for treatment.

9.3.2 Risk Factors

The principal risk factors for the development of CAC are [24, 25]:

– IBD diagnosis at young age (<15 years) and longer duration of the disease [13, 26]
– male sex
– extensive colitis
– persistence and severity of the inflammation: an important marker of disease severity and persistence of inflammation maybe the development of colonic strictures. Recent studies suggest that 2% to 3.5% of colonic strictures harbor dysplasia or colorectal cancer [13, 27, 28]—coexistence of PSC: it is considered a major risk factor for CRC in IBD patients, particularly those with UC. A study found that among a cohort of 101 CAC cases, nearly 20% ($n = 20$) had a concurrent diagnosis of PSC [15]. The risk of CRC is not affected by prior liver transplantation. Time to CRC onset was similar in patients with PSC and UC and those with UC alone, but the former group was five times more likely to develop CRC [26].

Focusing on CD-related risk factors, some studies identified an augmented risk among patients with small bowel-limited CD, but others demonstrated that most often there is a combination of those with both small and large bowel CD [21].

CD surgery still presents a challenge to both gastroenterologist and surgeon. The preservation of bowel length is important to maintain the digestive and absorptive functions of the gut. Strictureplasty has shown to be safe and effective, and its sites may be expected to have a similar rate of cancer development as unresected areas of CD because the inflamed area is left in place. Long strictureplasty (e.g., Finney-type procedures) also creates a short segment of excluded or bypassed intestine. Theoretically, this might have a potential to increase the likelihood of tumor formation [29, 30].

With regard to fistulating CD, fistula-related adenocarcinomas can arise in patients with long-standing perianal CD, and it may be associated with adenomatous transformation of the fistula tract epithelium. Early disease onset, disease duration exceeding 10 years, chronic colitis with high inflammatory activity, and persistence of chronic fistulas and stenosis seem to be associated with malignant transformation [31].

Regarding cancer risk in patients who underwent proctocolectomy with IPAA, a preoperative diagnosis of dysplasia or cancer of the colon or rectum is a risk factor for pouch dysplasia or adenocarcinoma. A Dutch registry study identified 25 cases of pouch neoplasia, including 16 adenocarcinomas, in 1200 IBD patients who had had IPAAs (1.83%). The risk was increased approximately fourfold in those with prior colorectal dysplasia and 25-fold in those with a history of CRC [26, 32].

9.3.3 Carcinogenesis

Different than sporadic CRC, which usually occurs as the endpoint of the adenoma–carcinoma sequence, the CRC correlated with CD and UC follows the sequence inflammation-dysplasia carcinoma [14].

Chronic inflammation and the degree of immunosuppression are the main driving factors for IBD-related carcinogenesis, which is a process of clonal evolution [12].

IBD-associated inflammation has the potential to mediate clonal evolution over time, by the following mechanisms: epithelial colonic cells suffer from genomic instability induced by oxidative stress, linked to chronic inflammation. Inflammatory infiltrate in UC generates oxygen radicals and nitrogen species (ROS and NOS), as well as chemokines and cytokines (IL-6, STAT3, TNF-α, IL-10, IL-12, and IL-23) that affect numerous metabolic processes involved in cell repair; therefore, this microenvironment provides a selective advantage to those clones able to more rapidly repopulate the healing mucosa and to survive a cytotoxic inflammatory insult (13, 34, 35].

A proper understanding of genetic mutations should allow a better stratification of IBD patients according to their risk for dysplasia and invasive carcinoma, in order to personalize their treatment and surveillance. Several studies have identified the tissue expression of specific proteins such as p53 and p21 in patients with IBD, in order to identify the natural evolution of these biomarkers and their relationship with carcinogenesis [33].

Actually, mutant clones frequently bear mutations in key tumor-suppressor genes including TP53 (encoding p53) and CDKN2A (encoding p16), in the proto-oncogene KRAS, and in the protein p2124–27 [12].

p53 is a tumor suppressor, regulating gene expression to prevent mutations of the genome and inducing apoptosis in case of DNA damage repair failure. It is the most frequently abnormal protein in human cancer. p21 is a cyclin-dependent kinase inhibitor, inducing growth arrest of cells with DNA damage, usually controlled by protein p53.

Both have demonstrated to be important biomarkers used to confirm dysplasia lesions. They also have prognostic significance; patients with significant and prolonged overexpression of p53 and p21 have a higher risk of developing dysplasia. Correlated overexpression of p53 and p21 in epithelial cells in UC indicates accumulation of cellular mutation triggered by oxidative stress and build-up of toxic products in stromal microenvironment of colonic mucosa [33].

Moreover, a recent study found that architectural distortion seems to be significantly correlated with p53 and p21 overexpression in epithelial cells. Thus, this histologic abnormality is a good parameter for evaluating the risk of degeneration in samples without dysplasia and compels a more careful endoscopic examination of mucosa especially in patients with long-standing disease. The immunohistochemical evaluation of p53 and p21 can be used as tissue biomarker for identification of patients with higher risk for dysplasia, diminishing the false-negative results [33].

A series of genes have been studies over the years. In particular, a large meta-analysis of individual-level data that included 11,794 cases of CRC and 14,190 controls, examined the association of GWAS-identified risk variants for UC and CD on risk of CRC. The (T) allele in rs11676348, a UC susceptibility locus located on chromosome 2, seems to be inversely associated with risk of CRC. In addition, using a subgroup of CRC cases with known histologic and molecular data, we showed that rs11676348 was particularly associated with lower risk of CRC tumors with Crohn's-like reaction, MSI-H status, and mucinous components which are characteristics of each tumor with high inflammatory burden. The allele rs11676348 was identified in GWAS of UC to be correlated with expression of CXCR2 gene. The CXCR2 gene is a member of G-protein-coupled receptor family with high affinity for IL-8 and primarily mediates migration of neutrophils to the site of inflammation and facilities the angiogenic effect of IL-8 in intestinal microvascular endothelial cells. More recently, CXCR2 has been implicated in development of CRCs associated with chronic colonic inflammation in experimental models [34, 35].

Several studies have demonstrated a higher incidence of MSI-H (Micro Satellites Instability) in the cancers that develop in the setting of long-standing UC with severe inflammation [36]. Specifically, compared with MSS stable tumors, MSI-H tumors are characterized by a higher inflammatory burden [36]. Moreover, it has been demonstrated that chronic inflammation is associated with an imbalance in base excision-repair enzymes that contributes to microsatellite instability [34].

Animal model studies demonstrate how transcription signaling by NF-κB, a master regulator of inflammation that has a key role in IBD pathogenesis, promotes the survival of premalignant epithelial clones. IBD-mediated inflammation also promotes β-catenin stability through aberrant PI3K-AKT and NF-κB signaling to further enhance canonical Wnt activity. Epithelial STAT3 signaling is also upregulated in active IBD [12].

CACs have increased mutation frequencies of various other intracellular and intercellular signaling molecules. Among the most notable mutations, IL-16, a gene encoding a chemoattractant cytokine that is overexpressed in IBD in an inflammation-dependent manner. IL-16 has a potential role in directly mediating inflammation and so it has been speculated that a gene mutation encoding this protein could provide a survival advantage in the inflamed bowel. Another noteworthy mutation is in RADIL, a gene encoding a modulator of Rho GTPase signaling in cell migration, which might provide a selective advantage in mucosal healing [12].

Genetic studies have also compared familial CRC and CAC with the hypothesis that variants in different genes may be associated with both cancers.

For example, p53 mutations (common to both CRC and CAC) appear to occur earlier in carcinogenesis in CAC, as these mutations are more commonly observed in colitis-associated dysplasia than among sporadic polyps [13, 37]. Mutations in APC and K-ras, which are known to occur much earlier within the adenoma–carcinoma sequence of sporadic colorectal cancer, are seen less frequently in colitis-associated colorectal cancer and are thought to arise much later in the dysplasia–carcinoma sequence where they promote NFkB-mediated cytokine secretion, neovascularization, and maintenance of tumor growth [13, 37, 38].

To date more than 40 loci have been associated with familial CRC, with many of the SNPs mapping to regions in strong linkage disequilibrium (LD) with members of the TGF-β signaling pathway highlighting an important role for TGF-β signaling in CRC. There is little overlap between known IBD and CRC loci in humans suggesting different etiologies to both diseases [37, 39].

Nevertheless, it has also been demonstrated that the genomes of CACs and sporadic CRCs in humans interestingly show broad similarities. Both bear a high frequency of TP53 alteration and mutations in the oncogenes KRAS, BRAF, PIK3CA, CTNNB1, and the tumor suppressors SMAD4 and FBXW7 are at relatively high, albeit slightly different, frequencies [12].

Remarkably, these cancer-associated mutations do not alone cause neoplastic growth as the mutations are detected in non-neoplastic tissue. These "key" mutations might be necessary but insufficient for tumor growth, or the phenotypic effects of these mutations are critically modulated by epigenetic and/or microenvironmental constraints present in non-neoplastic mucosa [12]. Actually, a comprehensive understanding of carcinogenesis in IBD should not be limited to the study of mutation generation and spread via the epithelial crypt stem cell niche, but should also include a concomitant analysis of the inflammatory stromal microenvironment. Therapeutic interventions that modulate cancer risk in IBD should also target these aberrant microenvironmental changes [12].

Emerging studies in the field of microbiome analysis are revealing the role of the gut microbiota and intestinal barrier function in tumorigenesis, and animal studies are beginning to shed some light onto the complex and dynamic interplay between the altered immune system, the aberrant gut microbiome and cancer development in IBD. Specifically, it was hypothesized that dysbiosis, and changes in population of microbial species including Fusobacterium nucleatum, Bacteroides or Prevotella, might enhance CRC progression by simultaneously regulating multiple signaling cascades which could lead to upregulation of proinflammatory responses, oncogenes, modulation of host immune defense mechanism, and suppression of DNA repair system [40–42].

9.3.4 Dysplastic Lesions [43]

IBD dysplastic lesions have had different denominations over the years.

The most common definition divided dysplastic lesions into two growth patterns: flat or raised/polypoid. Raised lesions were indicated as dysplasia-associated lesion or mass (DALM) if these lesions developed inside an inflamed area. DALMs were subclassified in adenoma-like or nonadenoma-like lesions depending on macroscopic characteristics. DALM adenoma-like lesions consisted in a well-circumscribed sessile or pedunculated polyp that was usually removed using routine endoscopic methods similar to those for sporadic adenomas. Nonadenoma-like DALMs included plaques, irregular nodules, and wide basis masses. These kinds of lesions were not usually candidates for endoscopic resection [14, 44].

Anyway, a subgroup of panelists, participating to the SCENIC Consensus Statement in 2015 developed a set of terms for colonoscopic findings in IBD surveillance to establish uniformity in communication [43].

Descriptive phrases, modified from the Paris Classification, were recommended for adoption (Tables 9.1 and 9.2).

Before this Consensus Statement, lesions were defined as dysplasia-associated lesion or mass (DALM), adenoma-like, and nonadenoma-like.

Anyway, the consensus stated that this terminology should be abandoned.

Moreover, specific endoscopic characteristics were added, with regard to their management.

Table 9.1 Terminology for reporting findings on colonoscopic surveillance of patients with inflammatory bowel disease (modified from Paris Classification [43])

Term	Definition
Visible dysplasia	Dysplasia identified on targeted biopsies from a lesion visualized at colonoscopy
Polypoid	Lesion protruding from the mucosa into the lumen ≥2.5 mm
Pedunculated	Lesion attached to the mucosa by a stalk
Sessile	Lesion not attached to the mucosa by a stalk: entire base is contiguous with the mucosa
Nonpolypoid	Lesion with little (<2.5 mm) or no protrusion above the mucosa
Superficial elevated	Lesion with protrusion but <2.5 mm above the lumen (less than the height of the closed cup of a biopsy forceps)
Flat	Lesion without protrusion above the mucosa
Depressed	Lesion with at least a portion depressed below the level of the mucosa
General descriptors	
Ulcerated	Ulceration (fibrinous-appearing base with depth) within the lesion
Border	
Distinct border	Lesion's border is discrete and can be distinguished from surrounding mucosa
Indistinct border	Lesion's border is not discrete and cannot be distinguished from surrounding mucosa
Invisible dysplasia	Dysplasia identified on random (non-targeted) biopsies of colon mucosa without a visible lesion

Table 9.2 Summary of recommendations for surveillance and management of dysplasia in patients with inflammatory bowel disease [43]

Detection of dysplasia on surveillance colonoscopy

1. When performing surveillance with white-light colonoscopy, high definition is recommended rather than standard definition (strong recommendation, low-quality evidence)
2. When performing surveillance with standard-definition colonoscopy, chromoendoscopy is recommended rather than white-light colonoscopy (strong recommendation, moderate-quality evidence)
3. When performing surveillance with high-definition colonoscopy, chromoendoscopy is suggested rather than white-light colonoscopy (conditional recommendation, low-quality evidence)
4. When performing surveillance with standard-definition colonoscopy, narrow-band imaging is not suggested in place of white-light colonoscopy (conditional recommendation, low-quality evidence)
5. When performing surveillance with high-definition colonoscopy, narrow-band imaging is not suggested in place of white-light colonoscopy (conditional recommendation, moderate-quality evidence)
6. When performing surveillance with image-enhanced high-definition colonoscopy, narrow-band imaging is not suggested in place of chromoendoscopy (conditional recommendation, moderate-quality evidence)

Management of dysplasia discovered on surveillance colonoscopy

7. After complete removal of endoscopically resectable polypoid dysplastic lesions, surveillance colonoscopy is recommended rather than colectomy (strong recommendation, very low-quality evidence)
8. After complete removal of endoscopically resectable nonpolypoid dysplastic lesions, surveillance colonoscopy is suggested rather than colectomy (conditional recommendation, very low-quality evidence)
9. For patients with endoscopically invisible dysplasia (confirmed by a GI pathologist) referral is suggested to an endoscopist with expertise in IBD surveillance using chromoendoscopy with high-definition colonoscopy (conditional recommendation, very low-quality evidence)

The term endoscopically resectable indicates that

1. distinct margins of the lesion could be identified
2. the lesion appears to be completely removed on visual inspection after endoscopic resection
3. histologic examination of the resected specimen is consistent with complete removal
4. biopsy specimens taken from mucosa immediately adjacent to the resection site are free of dysplasia on histologic examination

Macroscopic and microscopic (histologic) characterization is fundamental to assess the management of the lesions [45].

Histological classification of dysplasia in UC is on the basis of the study by Riddle et al. in which they described five categories: negative for dysplasia, indefinite for dysplasia, low-grade dysplasia, high-grade dysplasia, and invasive carcinoma [14, 46].

It is estimated that the annual rate of progression to CRC or to advanced neoplasia in patients with UC-Low-Grade Dysplasia under surveillance is approximately

0.8% (95% CI, 0.4–1.3) and 1.8% (95% CI, 0.9–2.7), respectively, and this rate may be variable depending on whether or not diagnosis of LGD was confirmed by an expert gastrointestinal pathologist. Concomitant PSC, invisible dysplasia, distal colonic location, and multifocal LGD are potential high-risk features associated with progression to advanced neoplasia [47].

Even though adenomatous lesions are more common, serrated lesions do not have to be neglected. In particular, a study by Rubio et al. found that serrated lesions exist in the inflammatory mucosa of IBD and are associated with a characteristic molecular profile, characterized by an early appearance of the BRAF mutation at the hyperplastic stage followed by microsatellite instability at the carcinoma stage. This study reported a high prevalence of serrated adenoma accounting for nearly 29% of the noninvasive dysplastic lesions arising in IBD carcinomas [48, 49].

9.3.5 Surveillance

9.3.5.1 Colic Disease
The goal of endoscopic surveillance is to reduce the morbidity and mortality of colitis-associated carcinoma by either detecting and resecting dysplasia or detecting CRC at earlier, potentially curable stages. A cohort study of 149 patients with IBD-associated CRC found a 100% 5-year survival of patients who were enrolled in a surveillance program compared with 74% in the non-surveillance group ($P = 0.042$). Of 30 patients with CRC-related deaths, only one patient died in the surveillance group compared with 29 in the non-surveillance group during the study period [8].

Clinical guidelines worldwide are primarily focused on UC follow-up and recommend surveillance colonoscopy to reduce CRC-related death.

Current American Gastroenterology Association (AGA) and American College of Gastroenterology (ACG) guidelines recommend surveillance every 1–2 years after 8–10 years duration of disease, with exception of yearly intervals in those with a family history of CRC in a first degree relative or active inflammation. Those with risk factors such as primary sclerosing cholangitis should have yearly surveillance starting at the time of diagnosis.

The British Society of Gastroenterology (BSG) and the European Crohn's and Colitis Organization (ECCO) also advocate initiating surveillance 8–10 years after diagnosis and offer additional guidance on surveillance intervals based on risk stratification.

In particular, patients are stratified in three risk categories; low-, medium-, and high risk, which corresponds to different ranges of surveillance, respectively, of 5 years, 2–3 years, and 1 year for low-, medium-, and high risk [50, 51]. The quantification of the risk varies according to risk factors, such as familiarity, extent of disease, or association with PSC.

Yearly surveillance: patients with moderate to severe active inflammation, history of stricture, dysplasia, primary sclerosing cholangitis, or family history of CRC in a first-degree relative aged <50 years old.

Surveillance every 2–3 years: patients with only mildly active inflammation, history of post-inflammatory polyps or family history of CRC (if no affected family members <50 years old).

Surveillance every 5 years: patients with only left-sided colitis or Crohn's colitis with <50% colon involved need surveillance colonoscopy only every 5 years. Notably, the recommended interval for surveillance for patients with extensive colitis but no active endoscopic and histologic inflammation is also 5 years [14, 52].

Several cost-effectiveness studies have been made over the years, confirming the cost-effectiveness of endoscopic surveillance. Rubenstein et al. [53] analyzed the cost-effectiveness of different surveillance strategies for men at age of 35 years with a 10-year history of UC. They considered two population subgroups, patients with and without medication of 5-aminosalicylates (5-ASA) and found surveillance in both to be cost-effective. In patients with 5-ASA, the most effective strategy under a willingness-to-pay threshold of $100,000 was colonoscopy surveillance every 3 years (ICER: $63,387 per quality-adjusted life years (QALY)). Without 5-ASA, the optimal strategy was annual colonoscopy (ICER: $69,105 per QALY). In the other study, Konijeti et al. [54] used chromoendoscopy and colonoscopy as surveillance tests. Both tests were cost-effective, but the analysis suggested that chromoendoscopy with targeted biopsies was superior than colonoscopy with random biopsies at all intervals.

The Negron et al. [55] study, which considered patients with IBD-PSC, also found that surveillance colonoscopy was cost-effective compared to no surveillance (for 2-yearly surveillance strategy the ICER of $37,522 per QALY was reported). In that study, annual surveillance was not cost-effective. (ICER: $174,650 per QALY).

Lutgens et al. [56] compared the cost-effectiveness of surveillance strategies of the American Gastroenterological Association (AGA) and the British Society of Gastroenterology (BSG) for patients with IBD. Although both strategies were equally effective, the BSG surveillance strategy was more cost-effective due to a lower number of colonoscopies (ICER: $11,130 per QALY) [57].

A number of biopsies and endoscopic technique have also been objective of study, as it is not always easy to endoscopically identify UC-associated CRC or dysplasia, as these lesions can be either invisible or very difficult to identify.

The most widespread technique for dysplasia surveillance in inflammatory bowel diseases is white-light endoscopy with random biopsies; however, some studies have questioned the diagnostic accuracy of white-light endoscopy, reporting a sensitivity of 76%, because dysplasia in flat mucosa can be difficult to detect. Therefore, the feasibility of this approach has been strongly challenged and the introduction of novel techniques has been encouraged [9].

At present, the guidelines recommend use of non-targeted biopsy (random biopsy) for surveillance colonoscopy, in which either 4 biopsy specimens for every 10 cm or >33 biopsy specimens are obtained. However, random biopsy has been recognized to be costly and time consuming and targeted biopsy has recently received much attention as an alternative. Studies have found that 61–84% of neoplastic lesions could be visualized by recent endoscopy techniques and, therefore, the guidelines suggest the possible use of targeted biopsy in place of random biopsy to improve the efficacy of surveillance. In targeted biopsy, specimens are obtained only when endoscopic findings indicate the possibility of neoplasia, leading to a smaller number of samples and resulting in a more cost-effective method. In a randomized controlled trial, we found that targeted and random biopsies detect similar proportions of neoplasias.

However, a targeted biopsy appears to be a more cost-effective method. Random biopsies from areas without any signs of present or past inflammation were not found to contain neoplastic tissues.

Recent guidelines recommend the use of a target biopsy; however, there has been no concrete evidence to show that a target biopsy should replace a random biopsy completely, and their effectiveness is comparable, while the cost-effectiveness is superior for target biopsies. When performing a targeted biopsy, it is recommended that a random biopsy sample be taken from the rectum. On the other hand, when performing a random biopsy, obtaining biopsy specimens from areas without any signs of present or past inflammation can be omitted, which can reduce the number of unnecessary biopsies and increase the efficacy of the random biopsy [43, 45, 58, 59].

In addition, the practice of obtaining biopsies around dysplastic lesions has also been questioned. A study demonstrated that dysplasia is detected in about 5% of biopsies collected from mucosa surrounding dysplastic lesions. This observation indicates that endoscopists accurately delineate the borders of dysplastic lesions during surveillance of patients with IBD. The lack of clinical consequences from routinely collecting biopsies from areas surrounding dysplastic lesions casts doubt on the usefulness and cost-effectiveness of this practice [50].

Overall, the application of guidelines about the correct number and type of biopsy during a surveillance colonoscopy is not yet optimal.

In Germany, only 9% of gastroenterologists follow the guidelines and in 50% of colonoscopies <10 biopsies are obtained. For this reason, in recent years attention is shifting from random biopsies to those obtained through the use of special endoscopic techniques, such as chromoendoscopy and other newer endoscopic techniques, such as endomicroscopy [14].

With the improvement of endoscopic equipment, the concept of IBD surveillance has been changing. Recent guidelines from the British Society of Gastroenterology (BSG) and the European Crohn's and Colitis Organization (ECCO) recommend targeted biopsy with panchromoendoscopy, especially when carried out by an experienced gastroenterologist [16, 43, 45, 59, 60].

The 2015 ASGE guideline now suggests chromoendoscopy as the preferred method, whereas random biopsies should only be used if chromoendoscopy is not technically feasible or not available [43, 45, 52, 59, 60].

It is important to underline that although guidelines are more often focused on UC surveillance, they are applicable to CD.

9.3.5.2 Surveillance in Case Fistulating, Strictures and After Surgery

Perianal fistulas occur in a significant portion of patients with Crohn's disease and often require repeat surgical treatment for abscess drainage or attempted repair of the fistula. As previously described, fistula-related adenocarcinomas can arise in patients with long-standing perianal CD, and it may be associated with adenomatous transformation of the fistula tract epithelium. Regular surveillance for anorectal carcinoma should be requested for all patients with perianal CD. It should include routine biopsy of any suspicious lesion and a biopsy under anesthesia or curettage of fistula tracts when needed.

Diagnosing dysplasia/cancer on endoscopic biopsies is a challenge in clinical practice, especially in the presence of strictures, and the absence of dysplasia or cancer on endoscopic biopsies cannot formally rule out the presence of dysplasia/cancer overall. Hence, the fear of missed colorectal cancer complicating colonic stricture leads frequently to colonic resection in these IBD patients [27].

In case of cancer or high-grade dysplasia (HGD) on colonic stricture, the decision must be the surgical resection; actually, colorectal strictures represent 2.3% of overall surgery indication in IBD [27].

Cancer development in the ileal pouch and the remnant rectum has been the concern after surgical resection for patients with ulcerative colitis (UC). Patients who underwent ileo-rectal anastomosis (IRA) are known to be at risk for the development of rectal cancer and require surveillance colonoscopy as those who have not received surgery [51]. It has been reported that the risk of postoperative neoplasia is lower in patients with UC receiving IPAA due to excision of the rectum than in those receiving IRA. However, cases of dysplasia/cancer have been reported even after IPAA [61].

IPAA has replaced IRA for most UC surgeries due to postoperative inflammation and the risk of neoplasia development in the remnant rectum with IRA. However, IRA has several advantages over IPAA in terms of anal and sexual functions and fecundity and thus, IRA is currently considered in selected cases, previously clarifying the risk of neoplasia development after IRA. There are no guidelines regarding surveillance after IRA, and the effectiveness of early detection of neoplasia is unclear.

IPAA is generally recommended for patients with UC based on the risk of cancer in the remnant rectum or ileal pouch. However, these results demonstrate that IRA with vigilant surveillance can be a viable alternative for those who hope to become pregnant or to preserve anal and sexual functions [61].

For patients who have had IPAA surgery, the development of dysplasia in either the ileal pouch mucosa or anorectal mucosa has been reported although appears to be rare.

Patients with a history of prior CRC, PSC, or refractory pouchitis should be considered for annual surveillance, with biopsies being obtained in the pouch as well as distally within the anal transition zone. Nevertheless, the ideal interval/need for continued surveillance for cancer developing in the pouch for patients without risk factors following an IPAA is still unknown [18].

ECCO endoscopy guidelines suggest that annual surveillance in such patients with high risk of pouch neoplasia may be worthwhile, at clinician discretion. If dysplasia is noted early after surgery, careful annual pouch surveillance is needed, with multiple biopsies of the ileal reservoir and the anorectal mucosa below the ileo-anal anastomosis [26].

9.3.5.3 Endoscopic Techniques

In recent decades, we have assisted to dramatic improvements in endoscopic devices, and several new techniques for enhancing and ameliorating the vision of the mucosa have appeared.

These techniques have been applied to surveillance colonoscopy for inflammatory bowel disease (IBD) patients [62, 63].

Among these: High Definition (HD) endoscopy; Magnification endoscopy (ME); Dye- and Virtual Chromoendoscopy (VCE); Confocal Laser Endomicroscopy (CLE); endocytoscopy (EC).

In patients undergoing surveillance with HD, Dye Chromoendoscopy (DCE), and VCE (but not White-Light Endoscopy (WLE)), current evidence supports DCE as the preferred method of surveillance [13], but there is less evidence regarding i-SCAN or newer narrow-band imaging (NBI) VCE techniques [64] (Table 9.3).

9.3.5.4 Magnification Endoscopy

Magnification endoscopy is performed by an endoscope with a variable lense, which allows to modify the magnification degree until 150-fold. Thanks to this feature that is possible to have a detailed characterization of the mucosal surface and the pit pattern. It has been shown that magnification endoscopy combined with chromoendoscopy has the potential to improve targeting biopsy examination in patients with long-standing colitis and facilitate early detection of intraepithelial neoplasia and colorectal cancer [44].

Full-spectrum endoscopy (FUSE) is a novel high definition endoscope that incorporates camera lenses to the right and left sides of the colonoscope tip in addition to the forward-viewing lens. These three lenses deliver a 330° panoramic field of view of the mucosa as opposed to the 170° field of view from a conventional forward-viewing colonoscope (FVC). Improved visualization of the side walls, blind spots, and behind folds significantly decreased adenoma miss rates from 41% using FVC (20 adenomas missed of a total of 49) to 7% using FUSE (5 adenomas missed of a total of 67) in a tandem back-to-back colonoscopy study of a non-IBD population. The total endoscopy times is similar between FVC (19.1 min) and FUSE (21.2 min; $P = 0.32$), but the colonoscope withdrawal time was significantly longer for FUSE (15.8 min) than FVC (12.0 min; $P = 0.03$). The mean dysplasia miss rate per subject remained significantly higher for FVC (0.83) than FUSE (0.19; $P < 0.0001$) when controlled for the longer withdrawal time for FUSE. Panoramic mucosal views obtained by three cameras may reduce dysplasia miss rates by visualizing lesions behind folds and in blind spots that are missed by a single forward-viewing camera. FUSE does not replace chromoendoscopy and the two techniques are complementary [65].

Table 9.3 Suggested steps for implementation of chromoendoscopy into endoscopic practice [43]

Equipment	
Colonoscope	High-definition colonoscope, monitor, and cables
Accessories	Apply dye via the following:
	Water jet channel by using water pump attached to the endoscope activated via foot pedal or spray catheter: length 240 cm, endoscope accessory channel 2.8 mm
Contrast agent	Indigo carmine, 5-mL ampule (0.8%)
Procedure and protocol	
Time allotment	Consider doubling colonoscopy time slot initially during the learning curve period
Standard operating procedure	Complete colonoscopy to cecum
	Lavage with water and suction during intubation
	Prepare dye solution during insertion for application via the foot pump or spray
	Indigo carmine (0.03%): mix 2 5-mL ampules of 0.8% indigo carmine with 250 mL water
	Methylene blue (0.04%): mix one 10-mL ampule of 1% methylene blue with 240 mL water
	If using a foot pump: once the cecum is intubated, the water irrigation can be exchanged with the contrast solution. Apply the dye solution in a circumferential technique while withdrawing the colonoscope. Direct spray to the antigravity side
	If using a spray catheter: the dye spray catheter is inserted into the biopsy channel; the catheter tip should protrude 2–3 cm from the endoscope. Apply dye solution segmentally by using a rotational technique while withdrawing the colonoscope to cover the surface mucosa with dye
	Suction any excess solution after approximately 1 min to aid mucosal visualization.
	Focus on 20–30-cm segments sequentially with insertion of the endoscope to the proximal extent of each segment before slow withdrawal and mucosal visualization
	Targeted dye spray for suspicious lesions:
	Prepare more concentrated dye solution for application
	Indigo carmine (0.13%): mix one 5-mL ampule of 0.8% indigo carmine with 25 mL water
	Methylene blue (0.2%): mix one 10-mL ampule of 1% methylene blue with 40 mL water
	Spray about 30 mL directly from a 60-mL syringe through the biopsy channel
	Remove endoscopically resectable suspicious lesions by using polypectomy or endoscopic mucosal resection
	Do targeted biopsies of any unresectable abnormality visualized through chromoendoscopy to diagnose dysplasia
	Do biopsies of flat area surrounding lesions to assess for dysplasia
	Consider tattoo of suspicious dysplastic lesions arising from flat mucosa or not amendable to complete removal
	Recommendations regarding the need to perform random, non-targeted biopsies for detection of dysplasia vary
	If biopsies for dysplasia are not done, two random biopsies in every bowel segment are commonly recommended to document microscopic disease activity

Reprinted from Laine, SCENIC consensus [43]

9.3.5.5 Chromoendoscopy

Chromoendoscopy is distinguished in dye-based (DBC) and dye-less imaging techniques (DLC).

Dye agents uses in DBC can be grouped into three types:

- Contrast agents (Indigo carmine and Acetic acid): they do not "stain" the colonic mucosa, but rather the dye pools in the grooves such that contrast visualizes subtle mucosal irregularities
- Absorptive agents (Toluidine blue, Lugol, Cresyl violet, and Methylene blue)
- Reactive staining agents (Congored and Phenol red): they stain the convex area of the colonic mucosa but not the grooves.

These agents are frequently used through spraying or catheters. Chromoendoscopy in combination with high magnification allows a better definition of spreading and degree of inflammation, if compared with standard white-light colonoscopy, in particular in patient with IBD. In addition, these techniques highly improve early detection of intraepithelial CRC [44].

Description of the Chromoendoscopy Technique

In selecting patients to undergo chromoendoscopy, it is important that the patients' disease activity is in remission and that they have good quality bowel preparation. Dye can be applied by various methods including spray catheter, flushing pumps, and recently as controlled released oral formulation taken with bowel preparation. Most clinical studies used spray catheters, but Picco and colleagues showed similar efficacy with the pump technique. A dilute dye solution (0.04% methylene blue or 0.03% indigo carmine) should be prepared to be compatible for use with the forward wash jet. Additionally, a 0.13% indigo carmine solution or 0.2% methylene blue solution should be prepared for use during lesion characterization.

During insertion, it is important to thoroughly wash and suction the mucosa to remove any residual stool and debris, which may hinder lesion detection during dye spraying. Once the cecum is reached, the water container should be exchanged for the dilute dye container. Dye should be sprayed toward the non-dependent mucosal surface for efficiency. This should be performed segmentally during withdrawal. Excess dye is suctioned to leave a thin layer of dye over the entire examined mucosa.

Careful inspection should then be performed with attention to areas that may be elevated, depressed, villous, and nodular in appearance or are friable or have an abnormal vascular pattern. Once a suspicious area has been identified, a 60 cc syringe of concentrated dye should be used to spray the mucosa directly through the working channel to allow improved characterization of visible dysplasia and margins [52].

Kiesslich et al. demonstrated the effectiveness of methylene blue-aided CE by applying Kudo's pit pattern diagnosis for UC surveillance in 2003 [21]. The study further investigated the usefulness of chromoscopy-guided endomicroscopy and showed a higher detection rate of neoplastic lesions using chromoscopy-guided endomicroscopy compared with conventional endoscopy in a RCT. However, the superiority of endomicroscopy over CE was not demonstrated.

A meta-analysis by Subramanian et al. investigated the usefulness of CE. CE resulted to be superior to conventional WLE regarding the dysplasia detection rate in both flat and raised lesions and the proportion of targeted biopsies although the examination time for CE was significantly longer than that for WLE. The usefulness of CE has been generally accepted [3].

Given these evidences, BSG and ECCO consensus guidelines on endoscopy in IBD recommend pan-colonic methylene blue or indigo carmine chromoendoscopy during surveillance colonoscopy, with targeted biopsies of any visible lesion. When chromoendoscopy is not available, multiple random biopsies should be performed [16, 44].

However, dye-based chromoendoscopy has some potential limitations, mainly its availability but especially the length of procedure. Moreover, dyes do not always coat all surface required and this procedure does not allow a detailed analysis of subepithelial capillary network, which is another important feature in the diagnosis of CRC [44].

DLC is grouped into optical chromoendoscopy and virtual chromoendoscopy.

Optical chromoendoscopy includes narrow-band imaging (NBI; Olympus®).

Virtual chromoendoscopy includes i-SCAN (Pentax®) and Fujinon intelligent color enhancement (FICE; Fujinon®).

NBI uses optical filters, applied on the light source of endoscope, which narrow the bandwidth of spectral transmittance. This methodology highly enhances the visualization of blood vessels pattern. It has been studied for CRC screening in IBD but has not been shown to be superior to white light or chromoendoscopy [52].

Efthymiou et al. compared NBI with CE and concluded that NBI was not superior to CE in the ability to detect dysplasia. Therefore, NBI is not yet recommended for routine UC surveillance in its present form. However, it may be useful for characterizing dysplastic lesions. For instance, it may be worthwhile to distinguish the tortuous pattern for any suspicious lesions in order to maximize the sensitivity of targeted biopsies, as NBI is an easily applied procedure which only requires the pressing of a button to change the mode if equipped [16, 66].

i-SCAN and FICE, instead, use digital postprocessing with computed spectral estimation to achieve a better tissue contrast, without using optical filters inside of the video endoscope.

FICE and i-SCAN use endoscopic images and reconstruct virtual images in real time by increasing the intensity of blue light to a maximum and by decreasing red light and green light to a minimum resulting in an improved contrast of the capillary patterns and enhancement of the mucosal surface.

To date, only a few studies have investigated the efficacy of FICE and i-SCAN for UC surveillance; therefore, they are not applied in every day practice [16, 44].

9.3.5.6 Confocal Endomicroscopy

Confocal laser endomicroscopy (CLE) is an endoscopic modality that was developed to obtain very high magnification of the mucosal layer of the gastrointestinal (GI) tract, and it has the potential to enable histological diagnosis in real time. CLE is based on tissue illumination using a low power laser and the subsequent detection of fluorescent light that is reflected back from the tissue through a pinhole. To obtain confocal images, exogenous fluorescence agents can be administered either topically or systemically. The most common topical contrast agents that are applied by a spraying catheter are acriflavine and cresyl violet, whereas the most widely used systemically administered fluorescent agent is intravenous fluorescein sodium. There are two types of CLE: endoscope-based (eCLE) and probe-based (pCLE) endomicroscopy. To perform eCLE, a dedicated endoscope with a miniaturized confocal scanner integrated into the distal tip is employed. The second system is pCLE (Cellvizio, Mauna Kea Technologies, Paris, France), which employs confocal miniprobes that are passed down the accessory channel of any standard endoscope, providing rapid microscopic image in real time.

The advantages of pCLE are its versatility and the possibility of combining it with other imaging modalities such as virtual chromoendoscopy or magnification.

CLE also demonstrated high applicability and superiority over standard endoscopy in the study of IBD. In particular, CLE can be used in the assessment of disease activity, in the prediction of relapse, and in the description of mucosal alterations such as epithelial gaps, all of which are useful toward enhancing the comprehension of new pathogenic features that develop in patients with IBD. However, costs, need of specifically trained personnel and length of the procedures, generally limit the use of CLE to selected cases [14, 44, 67, 68].

9.3.5.7 Endocytoscopy

Endocytoscopy is based on a contact light microscope which enables real-time visualization of cellular structures of the superficial epithelial layer in a plane parallel to the mucosal surface. Similarly to CLE, systems integrated into the distal tip of an endoscope (iEC) and probe-based (pEC) are available. The device provides ultrahigh magnification imaging from an optical sampling site of about 0.5 mm in diameter.

Endocytoscopy requires preparation of the mucosal layer with absorptive contrast agents like methylene blue or toluidine blue. The technique seems to be useful and safe for the examination of gastrointestinal mucosal surfaces and could recognize neoplasia in aberrant crypt foci and distinguish cancerous lesions from noncancerous ones. EC has demonstrated its efficacy in the assessment of inflammatory disease activity and differentiation of single inflammatory cells in patients with IBD, with a 100% concordance with histologic examinations [44, 68].

Compared with CLE, less data on the assessment of mucosal inflammation in IBD are available for EC.

The detection of colitis-associated neoplasia or cancer with EC has not been studied to date.

9.3.5.8 Surveillance: Future Perspectives

Recently, the use of stool-based surveillance has been considered for noninvasive screening. In particular, a multitarget DNA test, commercialized as Cologuard (Exact Sciences, Madison WI), assays mutant KRAS, methylated BMP3, and methylated NDRG4; it is based on the detection of CpG island methylation in human

DNA isolated from stool. Studies demonstrated that methylated gene markers BMP3, vimentin, EYA4, and NDRG4 showed a high discrimination between neoplastic and non-neoplastic tissue [69].

Several other studies have since been conducted to evaluate the potential of stool-based testing for colitis-associated colorectal cancer surveillance, but to date, no well-validated panels are available for routine clinical use in IBD, and further studies are needed to compare the effectiveness of this approach with currently accepted endoscopic standards [13].

9.3.5.9 Management of the Lesions: Resection Techniques and Surveillance

The decision of endoscopic vs. surgical management of dysplasia in colitis is based on endoscopic and histologic findings as well as patient-rated factors such as age, comorbidities, patient preferences, and other risk analysis [62, 70, 71].

Endoscopic resection is recommended for appropriate patients with endoscopically visible dysplastic lesions followed by surveillance colonoscopy 3–6 months, and then yearly.

Colectomy is reserved for patients who have endoscopically unresectable lesions or endoscopically invisible high-grade dysplasia despite chromoendoscopy examinations or multifocal dysplasia [43].

Accordingly with the SCENIC Consensus, endoscopically resectable polypoid and nonpolypoid lesions are considered separately because:

- uncertainty about the natural history and relative risk of CRC for polypoid and nonpolypoid dysplastic lesions in patients with IBD. Only recently, because of improvements in endoscopic imaging, nonpolypoid lesions have been identified regularly. Little is known about the natural history of nonpolypoid lesions although studies inpatients without IBD suggest that the molecular biology of nonpolypoid colorectal neoplasms may differ from that of polypoid colorectal neoplasms.
- differences between methods for endoscopic resection of polypoid and nonpolypoid lesions, being endoscopic resection of nonpolypoid lesions typically more difficult and often requiring advanced endoscopic skills.
- confidence that the lesion has been completely removed may be lower for nonpolypoid than for polypoid lesions

9.3.5.10 Endoscopically Visible Dysplasia

Endoscopic resection is recommended over colectomy for polypoid dysplasia and for nonpolypoid visible dysplasia. Though recent advances in endoscopic imaging have improved the recognition of nonpolypoid lesions in patients with IBD, their natural history and outcomes for complete endoscopic resection are less known. Simple polypectomy may not be adequate for complete resection of polypoid dysplasia.

A study by Blonski et al. found that among patients with endoscopically treated dysplastic lesions, almost 50% of the lesions had incomplete resection. Cold forceps or cold snare was predominantly used [72]. Therefore, it is of paramount importance to improve the endoscopic management of dysplastic lesions in colitis. If the lesion is assessed to be endoscopically resectable, it is necessary to use the proper technique with the aim to ensure complete endoscopic removal. Endoscopic mucosal resection (EMR) is the preferred method.

Hybrid endoscopic mucosal resection and endoscopic submucosal dissection (ESD) are other potential techniques, often determined by the lesion characteristics as well as the endoscopist's skills and experience [43].

Once resection is completed, biopsies of the adjacent area should be performed to document clearance. Additionally, the area should be tattooed to help facilitate surveillance. A history of dysplastic lesions, particularly nonpolypoid dysplastic lesions due to their flat shape and need for more advance dendoscopic resection techniques and large polypoid lesions >15 mm requiring EMR or ESD for resection, are a risk factor for CRC. Therefore, for these patients it is prudent to consider more frequent surveillance with the initial surveillance colonoscopy in 3–6 months.

For smaller polypoid lesions, postpolypectomy surveillance is recommended in 1 year [43, 52].

Dysplasia identified by random biopsy should be confirmed with chromoendoscopy as approximately 30% of patients may be found to have a lesion which may be amenable to resection. If no visible lesion is identified, management with endoscopic surveillance versus surgery can be individualized.

9.3.5.11 Endoscopically Invisible Dysplasia

Patient with endoscopically invisible low-grade dysplasia may be managed with intensive surveillance as risk of developing cancer is relatively low (14, 95% CI: 5–34 per 1000 patient years), while patients with endoscopically invisible high-grade dysplasia should consider colectomy. Confirmation of dysplasia by a pathologist with expertise in IBD is suggested before making management decisions.

For younger (aged <65 years) patients without comorbidity who have endoscopically invisible low- or high-grade dysplasia, colectomy may be a more clinically and cost-effective strategy [43, 52].

For patients with endoscopically invisible dysplasia (confirmed by a GI pathologist), referral is suggested to an endoscopist with expertise in IBD surveillance using chromoendoscopy with high definition colonoscopy [43, 52].

9.3.5.12 Chemoprevention and Protective Factors

Chemoprevention refers to the use of an anti-inflammatory therapy or other substance to reduce or prevent the development of cancer. The use of maintenance chronic ulcerative colitis therapies and notably the better control of inflammation by improved medical therapy and higher rates of mucosal healing could be important strategies for reducing CRC risk in UC patients. Intervening before the development of neoplasia might be a promising method to decrease cancer and prevent colectomy [73].

Literature data about the preventive effect of specific drugs on the development of CAC are scarce; moreover, the available studies are focused on the use of the first molecules used for the treatment of IBD, while long-term trials about the effect of new biologic therapies are awaited.

- *5-ASA and immunomodulators*: 5-ASA, the nuclear kappa-B pathway inhibitor, is a first-line agent for IBD therapy. This molecule is able to reduce oxidative stress, to inhibit cell proliferation and to promote apoptosis. Most reports indicated that 5-ASA reduces the risk of CRC in UC although literature data are controversial [18]. This protective effect has also been studied in CD, a study by Cahil et al. concluded that the use of salicylates is protective against SBA [21]. The protective effect of immunomodulators is primarily due to their role in the control of inflammation [74].
- *Ursodeoxycholic acid*: Ursodeoxycholic acid (UDCA) may be a practical chemoprevention against colonic exposure to bile acid inpatients with PSC. UDCA reduces the colonic concentration of the secondary bile acid as a carcinogen [18].
- *Steroids, aspirin, NSAIDs*: Although aspirin and other nonsteroidal anti-inflammatory medications have a chemopreventive effect in prevention of sporadic CRC, there are limited data in whether a similar effect is present in patients with IBD [13, 18].
- *Anti-TNF-alpha and biologic therapies*: Given the known importance of TNF and interleukins within the pathogenesis of colitis-associated colorectal cancer, more targeted inhibition of these pathways may offer an opportunity to prevent colitis-associated colorectal cancer, particularly among high-risk individuals who have developed early dysplastic lesions where these cytokines serve to stabilize the cancer microenvironment. Within colitis-associated colorectal cancer, although animal models have suggested that TNF antagonists may prevent the development or progression of dysplasia and cancer, and some population-based data within IBD have demonstrated a lower frequency of colorectal cancer among those treated with infliximab. Anyway, future studies regarding specific mutations related to CAC, will give the opportunity to find new therapeutic targets. For example, mutations in Rac GTP have been shown to be more common in IBD-associated neoplasia, and Rac1 inhibition has been shown in animals to prevent colorectal cancer carcinogenesis. The potential impact of such genetic observations is highlighted by a recent successful pilot trial against adenomas in patients with familial adenomatous polyps (FAP), where observations of EGFR upregulation in FAP-associated polyps led to a successful placebo controlled proof-of-concept human trial of erlotinib that markedly reduced adenoma burden and progression [13].

Total colectomy: The cumulative CRC risk in patients with UC is 30%–40% at 20–30 years after onset of disease, which might suggest that total colectomy is recommended after 15 years of disease in patients with UC. However, the role of prophylactic colectomy in patients with IBD remains controversial [18].

VITAMIN D: Over the years, more and more literature data have found that vitamin D is crucial for several biologic processes other than the regulation of bone metabolism. In particular, vitamin D has demonstrated to play a crucial role in autoimmune disease, as it controls immune cell trafficking and differentiation, modulated NK cell development, gut barrier function, antimicrobial peptide synthesis, and inflammation processes.

Regarding inflammation, studies showed that high levels of vitamin D may inhibit inflammation but lack of vitamin D does not accelerate or exacerbate the process, underlining how vitamin D can be intended to be a regulator of inflammation rather than a cause [75, 76].

Animal models of CAC showed a chemoprotective effect of vitamin D due to decreased colitis prior to tumor development [75, 77]. These data support the notion that vitamin D may be a beneficial adjunct therapy for IBD and CAC.

Other studies conducted on patients affected by colon, breast, and prostate cancer showed that almost a third of the patients were vitamin D deficient [75, 78].

Another mechanism through which vitamin D may protect against IBD is by improving intestinal epithelial barrier function. Patients with CD have increased intestinal barrier permeability which has been associated with inflammation and dysbiosis, as it results in increased exposure of the immune system to intestinal microbiota [76].

9.4   Extraintestinal Malignancies

The overall risk of extraintestinal cancer in patients with IBD is not increased relative to the general population. However, analysis by individual cancer sites shows that CD patients are more likely to develop cancers of the upper gastrointestinal tract, lung, urinary bladder, and non-melanoma skin cancers, and UC is associated with an increased risk of liver-biliary tract cancers and leukemia [26].

Nevertheless, extraintestinal malignancies related to IBD are mostly a consequence of immunosuppression.

Some hematological disorders and cholangiocarcinoma can be directly attributable to the presence of IBD.

9.4.1   Hematological Disorders

IBD patients show a trend toward higher risks of developing hematological malignancies. Compared with the general population, UC patients are significantly more likely to develop leukemia, whereas those with CD are at higher risk for lymphoma, especially non-Hodgkin lymphoma.

Early disease onset, male gender, and age >65 are risk factors for hematological malignancies in IBD patients. Inflammation and immune activation are involved in lymphogenesis; therefore, it can be speculated that inflammation plays a crucial role in hematological tumorigenesis, which in addition tends to affect organs where autoimmune responses occur [26].

Moreover, IBD have been associated to NOD2 gene. In particular, homozygote variants of the NOD2 gene predispose the carrier to CD, but they may also facilitate the development of hematological malignancies. Homozygotic carriers of the NOD2 variant rs2066847 are reportedly at higher risk for developing NHL and marginal zone lymphoma [79, 80].

9.4.2 Colangiocarcinoma

PSC is a chronic idiopathic disease with progressive fibrosing inflammatory destruction of intrahepatic and extrahepatic bile ducts and cholestasis. PSC has a male predominance and is frequently associated with inflammatory bowel disease (IBD).

PSC is typically progressive, with cirrhosis developing in the majority of patients within 10–20 years, and patients frequently require liver transplantation for survival. Additionally, patients are at increased risk of cholangiocarcinoma (CCA), which is a substantial cause of morbidity and mortality in this disease.

Cholangiocarcinoma develops in cholangiocytes which line the bile ducts, is highly aggressive, and has an overall poor prognosis. Therefore, in IBD patients with PSC, an adequate surveillance is noteworthy [81].

9.5 Cancer Surveillance due to Immunosuppression

Inflammatory bowel disease (IBD) relies on the use of immunosuppressant therapy to control disease activity and symptoms. These immunosuppressant treatments impair cell-mediated immunity, leading to a greater chance of opportunistic infections and neoplasia. Besides inherent disease-specific processes predisposing to cancers, the risk due to immunosuppressive therapy with corticosteroids, IMM, or anti-TNF agents reverses to baseline levels after discontinuation of these medications [82].

9.5.1 Hematological Malignancies

The overall risk of lymphoma among IBD patients (irrespective of medication use) has not been shown to be increased in several large population-based studies, but there is clear evidence that patients who are using thiopurines and antitumor necrosis factor agents are at increased risk of Non-Hodgkin Lymphoma [4, 83]. On the contrary, the overall risk of Hodgkin lymphoma in the IBD population remains low and comparable to non-IBD population [83].

Moreover, the risk is increased by the time of treatment duration: a study by Khan et al. demonstrated that the incidence rates of lymphoma during the first, second, third, and fourth year, and more than 4 years of thiopurine use were 0.9, 1.6, 1.6, 5, and 8.9/1000 person-years, respectively [22, 84]; the highest risk has shown to be in patients older than 50 years [85].

Regarding the type of lymphoproliferative disorder, the increased risk of lymphoma seems to be higher in patients with CD, whereas patients with both ulcerative colitis (UC) and CD are at an increased risk of developing leukemia [86].

Moreover, the risk is increased by Epstein-Barr virus infection, and most IBD patients who develop hematological malignancies after initiating thiopurine therapy are EBV-positive [26].

Risk of lymphoma among patients receiving anti-TNF therapy is elevated although also negative results have been published. In overall analysis, there was no difference in the frequency of malignancies between anti-TNF and control groups [22].

Studies conducted in pediatric age demonstrated that pediatric patients with IBD exposed to biologics in combination with thiopurines or thiopurines in the presence or absence of biologics have significantly increased risks of malignancy compared with the respective control populations.

These analyses confirm an association between thiopurines exposure and the development of malignancy, which previously has only been shown in adult studies. Consequently, it is noteworthy to weigh the potential benefits and risks of thiopurines in the treatment of pediatric patients with IBD, in a long-term perspective of surveillance [87].

9.5.2   Skin Malignancies

The risk of melanoma and NMSC (non-melanoma skin cancer) has been rising over several years in both IBD and non-IBD populations, and there is clear evidence of increased risk of melanoma in IBD patients with no significant change in time trend. The risk of NMSC is higher in patients using thiopurines compared with the non-IBD background population, with no significant change over time, and overall its risk has gone up in the last 15 years in IBD patients, likely because of increased use of thiopurines and antitumor necrosis factor agents [83].

It has been suggested that the increased risk of NMSC, most commonly squamous cell skin cancer, in IBD patients might be related to the use of both immunosuppressive medications and anti-TNF therapy, especially when used together with thiopurines [22].

Studies conducted on populations affected by rheumatoid arthritis have also shown that methotrexate is implicated in the augmentation of the risk for NMSC [88].

Data about IBD pediatric patients are limited, anyway a 2014 study conducted by Osterman et al. on pediatric CD patients did not find an increased incidence of malignancy in patients receiving adalimumab monotherapy compared with the expected incidence of NMSC or other cancers [89].

For what concerns melanoma, potential mechanisms of this increased risk in IBD patients include both underlying immune dysfunction resulting in altered tumor surveillance, and the use of immunosuppression medications. There have been conflicting data regarding the risk of melanoma with the use of tumor necrosis factor inhibitors, with some studies showing increased incidence with their use and others showing no increase compared with general population. A study by Long and colleagues [90] showed that the risk of melanoma was increased with biologics but not with immunomodulators. Another study performed by Peyrin-Biroulet et al. [91] did not detect any increase in the risk of melanoma in patients with IBD who were receiving thiopurines or antitumor necrosis factor treatment [83].

9.5.3   Cervical Cancer

The risk of cervical cancer does not seem to be increased in IBD in majority of studies, and the role of immunosuppression on the risk of cervical dysplasia in IBD is not clear. However, it is currently recommended that all women with IBD, particularly those on immunosuppressive therapy, take part in a screening program of cervical surveillance and undergo vaccination against HPV, if appropriate [22, 92].

Some investigators have shown an increased risk of cervical dysplasia among female, immunosuppressed IBD patients. The risk of anal dysplasia and cancer in this cohort has not been well studied [93].

9.5.4   Mouth Cancer

Mouth cancer is a major health problem. Multiple risk factors for developing mouth cancer have been studied and include history of tobacco and alcohol abuse, age over 40, exposure to ultraviolet radiation, human papillomavirus infection (HPV), nutritional deficiencies, chronic irritation, and existence or oral potentially malignant lesions such as leukoplakia and lichen planus.

An important risk factor for mouth cancer is chronic immunosuppression and has been extensively reported after solid organ transplantation as well as HIV-infected patients. Diagnosis of inflammatory bowel disease (IBD) is not yet considered as a risk factor for oral cancer development. However, a significant number of patients with IBD are receiving immunosuppressants and biological therapies which could represent potential oral oncogenic factors either by direct oncogenic effect or by continuous immunosuppression favoring carcinogenesis, especially in patients with HPV(+) IBD [94].

The effect of thiopurines (azathioprine, 6-mercaptopurine, and 6-thioguanine) on the development of mouth cancer is controversial. On the one hand, thiopurines may promote mouth carcinogenesis either by direct carcinogenic effect or by impaired function of immune cells. On the other hand, it has been suggested that topical AZA can be used for the management of oral immune-mediated inflammatory conditions and may allow control of oral symptoms. However, the long-term safety as well as the therapeutic potential of topical AZA as a mouth rinse vs. topical applications and the most effective and safe oral concentration of AZA still remains a challenge.

No studies about the effect of other drugs such as methotrexate, cyclosporine, tacrolimus, and glucocorticoids are reported.

Although current evidence suggests that anti-TNFs are not associated with an increased cancer risk in patients with IBD, there are reports in patients with other autoimmune diseases who developed mouth cancers during biological therapy [95, 96]. They have already been reported for years now in other groups of immunosuppressed patients.

Overall, it was demonstrated that patients with IBD belong to the high-risk group of developing mouth cancer lesions, and this could also be related to the increasing HPV prevalence [94].

References

1. Jussila A, Virta LJ, Pukkala E, Färkkilä MA. Malignancies in patients with inflammatory bowel disease: a nationwide register study in Finland. Scand J Gastroenterol. 2013;48:1405–13.
2. Jess T, Horváth-Puhó E, Fallingborg J, et al. Cancer risk in inflammatory bowel disease according to patient phenotype and treatment: a Danish population-based cohort study. Am J Gastroenterol. 2013;108:1869–76.
3. Kappelman MD, Farkas DK, Long MD, et al. Risk of cancer in patients with inflammatory bowel diseases: a nationwide population-based cohort study with 30 years of follow up. Clin Gastroenterol Hepatol. 2014;12(2):265–73.
4. Beaugerie L, Brousse N, Bouvier AM, et al. Lymphoproliferative disorders in patients receiving thiopurines for inflammatory bowel disease: a prospective observational cohort study. Lancet. 2009;374:1617–25.
5. Pasternak B, Svanström H, Schmiegelow K, et al. Use of azathioprine and the risk of cancer in inflammatory bowel disease. Am J Epidemiol. 2013;177(11):1296–305.
6. Duricova D, Fumery M, Annese V, et al. The natural history of Crohn's disease in children: a review of population-based studies. Eur J Gastroenterol Hepatol. 2017;29:125–34.
7. Peneau A, Savoye G, Turck D, et al. Mortality and cancer in pediatric-onset inflammatory bowel disease: a population-based study. Am J Gastroenterol. 2013;108:1647–53.
8. Bopanna S, Roy M, Das P, et al. Role of random biopsies in surveillance of dysplasia in ulcerative colitis patients with high risk of colorectal cancer. Intest Res. 2016;14(3):264–9.
9. Iannone A, Ruospo M, Wong G, et al. Chromoendoscopy for surveillance in ulcerative colitis and Crohn's disease: a systematic review of randomized trials. Clin Gastroenterol Hepatol. 2017;15(11):1684–97.
10. Adami H, Bretthauer M, Emilsson L, et al. The continuing uncertainty about cancer risk in inflammatory bowel disease. Gut. 2016;65(6):889–93.
11. Lutgens MW, van Oijen MG, van der Heijden GJ, Vleggaar FP, Siersema PD, Oldenburg B. Declining risk of colorectal cancer in inflammatory bowel disease: an updated meta-analysis of population-based cohort studies. Inflamm Bowel Dis. 2013;19(4):789–99.
12. Choi CR, Bakir IA, Hart AL, Graham TA. Clonal evolution of colorectal cancer in IBD. Nat Rev Gastroenterol Hepatol. 2017;14(4):218–29.
13. Dulai PS, Sandborn WJ, Gupta S. Colorectal cancer and dysplasia in inflammatory bowel disease: a review of disease epidemiology, pathophysiology, and management. Cancer Prev Res (Phila). 2016;9(12):887–94.
14. Fornaro R, Caratto M, Caratto E, et al. Colorectal cancer in patients with inflammatory bowel disease: the need for a real surveillance program. Clin Colorectal Cancer. 2016;15(3):204–12.
15. Jewel Samadder N, Valentine JF, Guthery S, et al. Colorectal cancer in inflammatory bowel diseases: a population-based study in Utah. Dig Dis Sci. 2017;62(8):2126–32. https://doi.org/10.1007/s10620-016-4435-4.
16. Hata K, Kishikawa J, Anzai H, et al. Surveillance colonoscopy for colitis-associated dysplasia and cancer in ulcerative colitis patients. Dig Endosc. 2016;28:260–5.
17. Han YD, Al Bandar MH, Dulskas A, et al. Prognosis of ulcerative colitis colorectal cancer vs. sporadic colorectal cancer: propensity score matching analysis. BMC Surg. 2017;17:28.

18. Sengupta N, Yee E, Feuerstein JD. Colorectal cancer screening in inflammatory bowel disease. Dig Dis Sci. 2016;61:980–9.
19. Kariv R, Remzi FH, Lian L, et al. Preoperative colorectal neoplasia increases risk for pouch neoplasia in patients with restorative proctocolectomy. Gastroenterology. 2010;139:806–12.
20. Scarpa M, van Koperen PJ, Ubbink DT, et al. Systematic review of dysplasia after restorative proctocolectomy for ulcerative colitis. Br J Surg. 2007;94:534–45.
21. Cahil C, Gordon PH, Petrucci A, Boutros M. Small bowel adenocarcinoma and Crohn's disease: any further ahead than 50 years ago? World J Gastroenterol. 2014;20(33):11486–95.
22. Nieminen U, Färkkilä M. Malignancies in inflammatory bowel disease. Scand J Gastroenterol. 2015;50:81–9.
23. Shwaartz C, Munger JA, Deliz JR, et al. Fistula-associated anorectal cancer in the setting of Crohn's disease. Dis Colon Rectum. 2016;59(12):1168–73.
24. Chen C, Neugut AI, Rotterdam H. Risk factors for adenocarcinomas and malignant carcinoids of the small intestine: preliminary findings. Cancer Epidemiol Biomark Prev. 1994;3:205–7.
25. Kaerlev L, Teglbjaerg PS, Sabroe S, Kolstad HA, Ahrens W, Eriksson M, Guénel P, Hardell L, Launoy G, Merler E, Merletti F, Stang A. Medical risk factors for small-bowel adenocarcinoma with focus on Crohn disease: a European population-based case-control study. Scand J Gastroenterol. 2001;36(6):641–6.
26. Annese V, Beaugerie L, Egan L, et al. European evidence-based consensus: inflammatory bowel disease and malignancies. J Crohn's Colitis. 2015:945–65.
27. Fumery M, Pineton de Chambrun G, Stefanescu C, et al. Detection of dysplasia or cancer in 3.5% of patients with inflammatory bowel disease and colonic strictures. Clin Gastroenterol Hepatol. 2015;13:1770–5.
28. Sonnenberg A, Genta RM. Epithelial dysplasia and cancer in IBD strictures. J Crohn's Colitis. 2015:769–75.
29. Menon AM, Mirza AH, Moolla S, Morton DG. Adenocarcinoma of the small bowel arising from a previous strictureplasty for Crohn's disease: report of a case. Dis Colon Rectum. 2007;50(2):257–9.
30. Collier P, Turowski P, Diamond DL. Small intestinal adenocarcinoma complicating regional enteritis. Cancer. 1985;55:516–21.
31. Gomollon F, Dignass A, Annese V, et al. 3rd European evidence-based consensus on the diagnosis and management of Crohn's disease 2016: part 1: diagnosis and medical management. J Crohns Colitis. 2017;11(1):3–25.
32. Derikx L, Kievit W, Drenth JP, et al. Prior colorectal neoplasia is associated with increased risk of ileoanal pouch neoplasia in patients with inflammatory bowel disease. Gastroenterology. 2014;146:119–28.
33. Popp C, Nichita L, Voiosu T, et al. Expression profile of p53 and p21 in large bowel mucosa as biomarkers of inflammatory-related carcinogenesis in ulcerative colitis. Dis Markers. 2016;2016:3625279.
34. Khalili H, Gong J, Brenner H, et al. Identification of a common variant with potential pleiotropic effect on risk of inflammatory bowel disease and colorectal cancer. Carcinogenesis. 2015;36(9):999–1007.
35. Jamieson T, Clarke M, Steele CW, et al. Inhibition of CXCR2 profoundly suppresses inflammation-driven and spontaneous tumorigenesis. J Clin Invest. 2012;122(9):3127–44.
36. Ishitsuka T, Kashiwagi H, Konishi F. Microsatellite instability in inflamed and neoplastic epithelium in ulcerative colitis. J Clin Pathol. 2001;54:526–32.
37. Van Der Kraak L, Gros P, Beauchemin N. Colitis-associated colon cancer: is it in your genes? World J Gastroenterol. 2015;21(41):11688–99.
38. Lennerz J, van der Sloot KW, Le LP, et al. Colorectal cancer in Crohn's colitis is comparable to sporadic colorectal cancer. Int J Color Dis. 2016;31:973–82.
39. Yaeger R, Shah MA, Miller VA, et al. Genomic alterations observed in colitis-associated cancers are distinct from those found in sporadic colorectal cancers and vary by type of inflammatory bowel disease. Gastroenterology. 2016;151:278–87.

40. Kumar A, Thotakura PL, Tiwary BK, Krishna R. Target identification in Fusobacterium nucleatum by subtractive genomics approach and enrichment analysis of host-pathogen protein-protein interactions. BMC Microbiol. 2016;16:84.
41. Yamamoto M, Matsumoto S. Gut microbiota and colorectal cancer. Genes Environ. 2016;38:11.
42. Kanauchi O, Mitsuyama K, Andoh A. The new prophylactic strategy for colitic cancer in inflammatory bowel disease by modulating microbiota. Scand J Gastroenterol. 2013;48:387–400.
43. Laine L, Kaltenbach T, Barkun A, et al. SCENIC international consensus statement on surveillance and management of dysplasia in inflammatory bowel disease. Gastroenterology. 2015;148:639–51.
44. Gabbani T, Manetti N, Bonanomi AG, et al. New endoscopic imaging techniques in surveillance of inflammatory bowel disease. World J Gastrointest Endosc. 2015;7(3):230–6.
45. Magro F, Gionchetti P, Eliakim R, et al. Third European evidence-based consensus on diagnosis and management of ulcerative colitis. Part 1: definitions, diagnosis, extra-intestinal manifestations, pregnancy, cancer surveillance, surgery, and ileo-anal pouch disorders. J Crohns Colitis. 2017;11(6):649–70.
46. Riddell RH, Goldman H, Ransohoff DF, Appelman HD, Fenoglio CM, Haggitt RC, Ahren C, Correa P, Hamilton SR, Morson BC, et al. Dysplasia in inflammatory bowel disease: standardized classification with provisional clinical applications. Hum Pathol. 1983;14(11):931–68.
47. Fumery M, Dulai PS, Gupta S, et al. Incidence, risk factors, and outcomes of colorectal cancer in patients with ulcerative colitis with low-grade dysplasia: a systematic review and meta-analysis. Clin Gastroenterol Hepatol. 2017;15:665–74.
48. Rubio CA, Befrits R, Jaramillo E, Nesi G, Amorosi A. Villous and serrated adenomatous growth bordering carcinomas in inflammatory bowel disease. Anticancer Res. 2000;20(6C):4761–4.
49. Iacucci M, Hassan C, Fort Gasia M, et al. Serrated adenoma prevalence in inflammatory bowel disease surveillance colonoscopy, and characteristics revealed by chromoendoscopy and virtual chromoendoscopy. Can J Gastroenterol Hepatol. 2014;28(11):589–94.
50. Ten Hove JR, Mooiweer E, Dekker E, et al. Low rate of dysplasia detection in mucosa surrounding dysplastic lesions in patients undergoing surveillance for inflammatory bowel diseases. Clin Gastroenterol Hepatol. 2017;15:222–8.
51. Hata K, Watanabe T, Kazama S, et al. Earlier surveillance colonoscopy program improves survival in patients with ulcerative colitis associated colorectal cancer: results of a 23-year surveillance program in the Japanese population. Br J Cancer. 2003;89:1232–6.
52. Yu JX, East JE, Kaltenbach T. Surveillance of patients with inflammatory bowel disease. Best Pract Res Clin Gastroenterol. 2016;30(6):949–58.
53. Rubenstein JH, Waljee AK, Jeter JM, Velayos FS, Ladabaum U, Higgins PD. Cost effectiveness of ulcerative colitis surveillance in the setting of 5-aminosalicylates. Am J Gastroenterol. 2009;104(9):2222–32.
54. Konijeti GG, Shrime MG, Ananthakrishnan AN, Chan AT. Cost-effectiveness analysis of chromoendoscopy for colorectal cancer surveillance in patients with ulcerative colitis. Gastrointest Endosc. 2014;79(3):455–65.
55. Negron ME, Kaplan GG, Barkema HW, Eksteen B, Clement F, Manns BJ, et al. Colorectal cancer surveillance in patients with inflammatory bowel disease and primary sclerosing cholangitis: an economic evaluation. Inflamm Bowel Dis. 2014;20(11):2046–55.
56. Lutgens M, van Oijen M, Mooiweer E, van der Valk M, Vleggaar F, Siersema P, et al. A risk-profiling approach for surveillance of inflammatory bowel disease-colorectal carcinoma is more cost-effective: a comparative cost-effectiveness analysis between international guidelines. Gastrointest Endosc. 2014;80(5):842–8.
57. Omidvari A. Cost effectiveness of surveillance for GI cancers. Best Pract Res Clin Gastroenterol. 2016;30:879–91.
58. Kornbluth A, Sachar DB. Ulcerative colitis practice guidelines in adults: American College of Gastroenterology, Practice Parameters Committee. Am J Gastroenterol. 2010;105:501–23; quiz 524.
59. Watanabe T, Ajioka Y, Mitsuyama K, et al. Comparison of targeted vs random biopsies for surveillance of ulcerative colitis-associated colorectal cancer. Gastroenterology. 2016;151:1122–30.

60. Mowat C, Cole A, Windsor A, et al. Guidelines for the management of inflammatory bowel disease in adults. Gut. 2011;60:571–607.
61. Ishii H, Hata K, Kishikawa J, et al. Incidence of neoplasias and effectiveness of postoperative surveillance endoscopy for patients with ulcerative colitis: comparison of ileorectal anastomosis and ileal pouch anal anastomosis. World J Surg Oncol. 2016;14:75.
62. Itzkowitz SH, Present DH, Crohn's and Colitis Foundation of America Colon Cancer in IBD Study Group. Consensus conference: colorectal cancer screening and surveillance in inflammatory bowel disease. Inflamm Bowel Dis. 2005;11:314–21.
63. Bernstein CN, Shanahan F, Weinstein WM. Are we telling patients the truth about surveillance colonoscopy in ulcerative colitis? Lancet. 1994;343:71–4.
64. Gasia MF, Ghosh S, Panaccione R, et al. Targeted biopsies identify larger proportions of patients with colonic neoplasia undergoing high-definition colonoscopy, dye chromoendoscopy, or electronic virtual chromoendoscopy. Clin Gastroenterol Hepatol. 2016;14:704–12.
65. Leong RW, Ooi M, Corte C, et al. Full-spectrum endoscopy improves surveillance for dysplasia in patients with inflammatory bowel diseases. Gastroenterology. 2017;152:1337–44.
66. Efthymiou M, Allen PB, Taylor AC, et al. Chromoendoscopy versus narrow band imaging for colonic surveillance in inflammatory bowel disease. Inflamm Bowel Dis. 2013;19:2132–8.
67. Fugazza A, Gaiani F, Carra MC, et al. Confocal laser endomicroscopy in gastrointestinal and pancreatobiliary diseases: a systematic review and meta-analysis. Bio Med Res Int. 2016;2016:4638683.
68. Tontini GE, Rath T, Neumann H. Advanced gastrointestinal endoscopic imaging for inflammatory bowel diseases. World J Gastroenterol. 2016;22(3):1246–59.
69. Kisiel JB, Konijeti GG, Piscitello AJ, et al. Stool DNA analysis is cost-effective for colorectal cancer surveillance in patients with ulcerative colitis. Clin Gastroenterol Hepatol. 2016;14:1778–87.
70. Picco MF, Pasha S, Leighton JA, et al. Procedure time and the determination of polypoid abnormalities with experience: implementation of a chromoendoscopy program for surveillance colonoscopy for ulcerative colitis. Inflamm Bowel Dis. 2013;19:1913–20.
71. Moussata D, Allez M, Cazals-Hatem M, et al. Are random biopsies still useful for the detection of intraepithelial neoplasia in IBD patients undergoing surveillance colonoscopy with chromoendoscopy? Gut. 2012;61(suppl 3):A24.
72. Blonksi W, Kundu R, Lewis J, et al. Is dysplasia visible during surveillance colonoscopy in patients with ulcerative colitis? Scand J Gastronterol. 2008;43:698–703.
73. Yashiro M. Ulcerative colitis-associated colorectal cancer. World J Gastroenterol. 2014;20(44):16389–97.
74. Gong J, Zhu L, Guo Z, Li Y, Zhu W, Li N, et al. Use of thiopurines and risk of colorectal neoplasia in patients with inflammatory bowel diseases: a meta-analysis. PLoS One. 2013;8:e81487.
75. Meeker S, Seamons A, Paik J, Treuting PM, Brabb T, Grady WM, Maggio-Price L. Increased dietary vitamin D suppresses MAPK signaling, colitis, and colon cancer. Cancer Res. 2014;74:4398–408.
76. Seamons A, Maggio-Price L, Paik J. Protective links between vitamin D, inflammatory bowel disease and colon cancer. World J Gastroenterol. 2016;22(3):933–48.
77. Hummel DM, Thiem U, Höbaus J, Mesteri I, Gober L, Stremnitzer C, Graça J, Obermayer-Pietsch B, Kallay E. Prevention of preneoplastic lesions by dietary vitamin D in a mouse model of colorectal carcinogenesis. J Steroid Biochem Mol Biol. 2013;136:284–8.
78. Ananthakrishnan AN, Cheng SC, Cai T, Cagan A, Gainer VS, Szolovits P, Shaw SY, Churchill S, Karlson EW, Murphy SN, Kohane I, Liao KP. Association between reduced plasma 25-hydroxy vitamin D and increased risk of cancer in patients with inflammatory bowel diseases. Clin Gastroenterol Hepatol. 2014;12:821–7.
79. Latella G, Rogler G, Bamias G, et al. Results of the 4th scientific workshop of the ECCO [I]: pathophysiology of intestinal fibrosis in IBD. J Crohns Colitis. 2014;8:1147–65.
80. Wilson J, Furlano RI, Jick SS, Meier CR. A population-based study examining the risk of malignancy in patients diagnosed with inflammatory bowel disease. J Gastroenterol. 2016;51:1050–62.

81. Horsley-Silva JL, Rodriguez EA, Franco DL, Lindor KD. An update on cancer risk and surveillance in primary sclerosing cholangitis. Liver Int. 2017;37(8):1103–9.
82. Yadav S, Singh S, Harmsen WS, et al. Effect of medications on risk of cancer in patients with inflammatory bowel diseases: a population-based cohort study from Olmsted County, Minnesota. Mayo Clin Proc. 2015;90(6):738–46.
83. Garg S, Loftus EV Jr. Risk of cancer in inflammatory bowel disease: going up, going down, or still the same? Curr Opin Gastroenterol. 2016;32:274–81.
84. Khan N, Abbas AM, Lichtenstein GR, Loftus EV Jr, Bazzano LA. Risk of lymphoma in patients with ulcerative colitis treated with thiopurines: a nationwide retrospective cohort study. Gastroenterology. 2013;145:1007–15.
85. Kotlyar DS, Lewis JD, Beaugerie L, et al. Risk of lymphoma in patients with inflammatory bowel disease treated with azathioprine and 6-mercaptopurine: a meta-analysis. Clin Gastroenterol Hepatol. 2015;13:847.
86. Madanchi M, Zeitz J, Barthel C, et al. Malignancies in patients with inflammatory bowel disease: a single-centre experience. Digestion. 2016;94:1–8.
87. Hyams JS, Dubinsky MC, Baldassano RN, et al. Infliximab is not associated with increased risk of malignancy or hemophagocytic lymphohistiocytosis in pediatric patients with inflammatory bowel disease. Gastroenterology. 2017;152(8):1901–1914.e3.
88. Scott FI, Mamtani R, Brensinger CM, et al. Risk of nonmelanoma skin cancer associated with the use of immunosuppressant and biologic agents in patients with a history of autoimmune disease and nonmelanoma skin cancer. JAMA Dermatol. 2016;152(2):164–72.
89. Osterman MT, Sandborn WJ, Colombel JF, et al. Increased risk of malignancy with adalimumab combination therapy, compared with monotherapy, for Crohn's disease. Gastroenterology. 2014;146:941–9.
90. Long MD, Martin CF, Pipkin CA, et al. Risk of melanoma and non-melanoma skin cancer among patients with inflammatory bowel disease. Gastroenterology. 2012;143:390–9.
91. Peyrin-Biroulet L, Chevaux JB, Bouvier AM, et al. Risk of melanoma in patients who receive thiopurines for inflammatory bowel disease is not increased. Am J Gastroenterol. 2012;107:1443–4.
92. Rivera-Acosta J, Aponte M, Villamil I, et al. Human papilloma virus awareness among hispanic females with inflammatory bowel disease. J Racial Ethnic Health Disparities. 2016;3:55–62.
93. Shah SB, Pickham D, Araya H, et al. Prevalence of anal dysplasia in patients with inflammatory bowel disease. Clin Gastroenterol Hepatol. 2015;13:1955–61.
94. Giagkou E, Christodoulou DK, Katsanos KH. Mouth cancer in inflammatory bowel diseases. Oral Dis. 2016;22:260–4.
95. Rousseau A, Taberne R, Siberchicot F, Fricain JC, Zwetyenga N. Cancer of the cheek in a patient under etanercept. Rev Stomatol Chir Maxillofac. 2009;110:306–8.
96. Antoniou C, Dessinioti C, Vergou T, et al. Sequential treatment with biologics: switching from efalizumab to etanerceptin 35 patients with high-need psoriasis. J Eur Acad Dermatol Venereol. 2010;24:1413–20.

Conclusions

10

Luigi Dall'Oglio

During my school in medicine, I was as an intern in one of the adult's surgical departments in Rome, where many patients with ulcerative colitis and Crohn's disease were treated. The only available endoscopic tool was the rigid rectoscopy, performed by surgeons.

Despite this important diagnostic limitation, I could observe and learn the correct clinical approach to these complex patients: full medical evaluation, radiological and rectoscopic pictures were evaluated and discussed between surgical and medical staff together with radiologists and overall histopathologists. Indeed, it was clear very early that histopathologist had a strategic role, in the side of the endoscopic and clinical staff, for correct diagnosis and evolution of the disease during the treatment.

This innovative approach for these complex patients was rarely used because of the rigid separation of surgical and medical environments.

The advent of flexible endoscopy, in Italy in the surgical units, step by step improved the diagnostic tools together with the medical and surgical/endoscopic collaboration. The endoscopic support in the diagnosis, treatment evaluation, and follow-up was always of strategic importance. It was progressively clear that IBD care is not possible without endoscopy.

The goal of mucosal healing, not only in ulcerative colitis but also in Crohn's disease, represented another specific indication for endoscopic evaluation.

When in 1977 I started pediatric flexible endoscopy, we were surprised to find IBD in adolescents, in children, and also in small children.

In our medical-surgical unit, endoscopy is the common denominator of all members—pediatric surgeons and gastroenterologists—and IBD is one of the most commonly followed and studied disease. I still would like to teach and share with my staff this goal: endoscopy is a tool for learning, studying, diagnosing, and

L. Dall'Oglio
Digestive Surgery and Endoscopic Unit, Bambino Gesù Children's Hospital, Rome, Italy
e-mail: dalloglio@opgb.net

© Springer International Publishing AG, part of Springer Nature 2018
L. Dall'Oglio, C. Romano (eds.), *Endoscopy in Pediatric Inflammatory Bowel Disease*,
https://doi.org/10.1007/978-3-319-61249-2_10

sometimes treating IBD patients; it must be strictly performed from the indications and the technique up to the prevention and management of complications. Everyone who performs endoscopy in IBD, regardless of medical or surgical extraction, must know the pathology and how to follow all the patients.

Everybody knows the evolution of pediatric IBD care: new diagnosis, new therapeutic strategies, and the opportunity of routine endoscopic evaluation of the therapeutic effects on the intestinal mucosa, as well as the innovative studies of immunology and microbiology on gut biopsies. Modern endoscopes and new sedation strategies, like the deep sedation, are now available for all the pediatric ages to improve the opportunity of correct diagnosis and follow-up.

Ileoscopic evaluation, either with videocapsule and enteroscopes, represented two endoscopic tools of fundamental importance for correct diagnosis in these difficult diseases.

At the moment, as it is clearly showed in this book, there is the opportunity to perform an endoscopic and histologic evaluation of all the intestinal mucosa: upper endoscopy, colon-ileo endoscopy, and full enteroscopy.

The different interpretation of the endoscopic pictures could represent an important limitation and so it is very important that indication to the different endoscopic maneuvers, bowel cleaning, exam conduction, and specimens collection must follow the published guide lines.

Adult endoscopic scientific societies improved the standardization of endoscopic maneuvers and, overall, the macroscopic descriptions of the gastrointestinal wall. This aspect is very important to standardize the correlation between clinical and endoscopic pictures.

It is also of fundamental importance that the one who perform the endoscopic maneuvers should also be the one who is involved in the clinical evolution of the patient and he should enter in the choice of the therapeutic strategy.

In case of adult endoscopist involved in the children's diagnostic procedures, it is mandatory the presence of the pediatric gastroenterologist in the endoscopic suite; otherwise he will never can have the full and proper knowledge of his patient.

Endoscopy currently allows to investigate immune analysis of the intestinal mucosa (i.e., routine histology, phenotyping of the lamina propria mononuclear cells by flow cytometry, and intracellular cytokine concentration), important scientific field of interest in worldwide.

Through endoscopy, there is the great chance to study the intestinal microbiota that has been well documented and implicated in the pathogenetic factors of IBD, together with genetic predisposition and immune system dysregulation. Recent evidence has demonstrated that modulation of gut microbiota is achievable through fecal microbiota transplantation (FMT). The efficacy of this treatment has been described for *Clostridium difficile* infection and IBD in adult patients. The pediatric experience is limited, but there is increasing interest in this therapeutic strategy, performed by endoscopy that allows a deep jejunal or cecal microbiota infusion.

Endoscopy has a great role in screening and colon cancer surveillance of long-standing IBD patients and in patients with concurrent diagnosis of primary sclerosing cholangitis (PSC): chromoendoscopy (methylene blue or indigo carmine) increases the sensitivity of standard endoscopy for the detection of dysplasia, guiding targeted biopsies.

ERCP therapeutic procedures treat the biliary tree PSC strictures, like a bridge treatment for liver transplant.

Therapeutic endoscopy represents an important tool in IBD-complicated patients; stricturing Crohn's disease and stenotic surgical anastomosis in every site of small intestine and colon could need endoscopic dilations that are useful to maintain bowel length avoiding the short gut syndrome. Endoscopic balloon dilation with standard colonoscopy or with mono-double balloon enteroscopy can be performed and repeated safely with minimal complications in IBD patients with good results.

In conclusion, endoscopy can help diagnosis and management of IBD patients in different ways. It will be interesting to understand the real role of endoscopic mucosal healing as an endpoint for medical therapy and in postoperative evaluations. However, endoscopy remains an excellent tool that will never replace the reasoning, intuition, and empathy of the physician who takes care of IBD patients.

Gastrointestinal endoscopy in IBD, improved by high level of technical and clinical training, should be at the center of IBD scientists' heart to reach a unit and well-documented management of the disease.